Online and
Personal

The reality *of* Internet relationships

Jo Lamble & Sue Morris

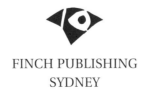

FINCH PUBLISHING
SYDNEY

Online and Personal: The reality of Internet relationships

This edition first published in 2001 in Australia and New Zealand
by Finch Publishing Pty Limited, ABN 49 057 285 248,
PO Box 120, Lane Cove, NSW 1595, Australia.

04 03 02 01   8 7 6 5 4 3 2 1

National Library of Australia
Cataloguing-in-Publication entry

Lamble, Jo.

Online and personal: the reality of internet relationships.

Bibliography.
Includes index.
ISBN 1 876451 17 3.

1. Internet (Computer network) – Social aspects.
2. Interpersonal relationships. I. Morris, Sue. II. Title.

303.4834

Edited by Marie-Louise Taylor
Text designed and typeset in Utopia by *Di∧gn*
Cover design by *Di∧gn*
Cover illustration by Andrew Bell
Printed by Brown Prior Anderson

Cartoons: The cartoons are reproduced with the permission of The Cartoon Bank/Scoop Media, Sydney and are copyrighted by those organisations and the individual illustrators: M. Stevens (page 18), J. Ziegler (pages 51 and 175), R. Mankoff (page 93) and M. Crawford (page 133).

Notes: The 'Authors' notes' at the back of this book contain useful additional information and references to quoted material in the text. Each reference is linked to the text by its relevant page number and an identifying line entry.

Disclaimer: The stories told in *Online and Personal* have been collected from a variety of sources. Some are based on real case studies, others are from people who agreed to be interviewed or who contacted us because they wanted their story told. Names and personal details have been changed to protect people's privacy. The chat room dialogues in the book were inspired by real chat room conversations, but the characters and dialogue content are fictional. Any resemblance to actual people or events is coincidental. While this publication outlines a number of strategies to assist the reader, it is not intended to serve as a replacement for psychological advice. The authors and publisher specifically disclaim any and all liability arising directly or indirectly from the use or application of any information contained in this book. If expert counselling is required, the services of a competent professional should be sought.

Contents

Foreword

Online and Personal is a thoughtful, thought-provoking book that will be a great help to anyone who uses or considers using the Net for business or pleasure.

Regardless of your degree of immersion in Net-affairs, Net-nooky or Net-working, this book provides crucial insights that will assist you in formulating an ethical, safe and maximally rewarding approach to your Net-adventures.

Make the most of your online relationships and enjoy the Net without sabotaging your existing relationships. Protect your kids from potential hazards and abuse. Formulate a 'netiquette' you can practise and be proud of, tailored to your own values and needs. Be aware of and guard against Net-addiction and Net-abuse. And most importantly, acknowledge that knowing how to get OFFline can be just as important as knowing how to get online. ***Online and Personal*** covers (and uncovers) all of these issues as well as providing invaluable insights into non-Net, real-life relationships. All this with a delicious sprinkling of humour.

I've revealed intimate and personal information to virtual strangers in emails of over a thousand words. I've hurled vitriolic emails that must have set the recipients' screens ablaze ... possibly provoked by little more than a misunderstanding. All kinds of things I'd have hesitated to do in real life, I've recklessly done, and regretted, in my virtual Net-reality.

The best thing about email is the instantaneous ease of sending. The beast of it is, once you press 'SEND' you can't retrieve it – even when your head has cooled and cleared and you have beat it mercilessly against a brick wall while wailing with the excruciating pain of remorse.

As a current user and past abuser (never again, Jo and Sue, I promise) of Internet technology, it was a huge relief to read **Online and Personal**. If only I'd read it *before* I got online. Oh well, it's never too late.

Dr Cindy Pan MBBS, FRACGP
General Practitioner, Television Poseur
and author of **Pandora's Box**.

About this book

Online and Personal came about by accident. We had just released *Side by Side: How to think differently about your relationship,* where we introduced our readers to the dangers associated with forming an Internet relationship if they were in a committed relationship. The overwhelming interest in this topic suggested there was a need for a book about how the Internet was affecting people's lives in general and their relationships in particular.

In *Online and Personal* we discuss the impact the Internet is having on people's personal lives. We look at those whose existing relationships are being threatened by Internet liaisons, single people who use the Net to meet people, others who feel their online behaviour is out of control, and what needs to be done to help children who go online. Given the Internet is a relatively new phenomenon in the average family home, there is still much to learn about how it affects us psychologically and what we need to do to moderate its influence.

Our ideas have been gathered from a variety of sources including our individual clients, our colleagues, family and friends, and from many people who agreed to be interviewed for the book. Indeed, that you are reading *Online and Personal* is testament to the fact that the Internet is a wonderful communication tool because when we started writing Sue moved to the US. We would not have been able to write this book as quickly and easily without the Internet. Being so reliant on the Internet has also opened our eyes to its downside. It was often agonisingly painful to type our thoughts in emails when we normally would have tossed around the ideas over lunch in the office. The time difference also added to our frustration, as we had to contend with sending an email full of ideas only to wait 24 hours until we received feedback. But nonetheless, we would say that writing a book about the Internet over the Internet has been a fabulous experience. We certainly have learnt a lot.

Online and Personal includes stories from Internet users in Australia and the US, input from our training as clinical psychologists, and techniques and exercises based on the psychological treatment model known as Cognitive Behaviour Therapy, developed by A. Beck and A. Ellis. These exercises are boxed and marked with a 'personal' icon throughout the book. We also make a number of suggestions about what you may need to do to protect yourself, your relationships and your children from the dangers of the Internet. If you are single and have met someone online, we look at what steps you can take to maximise the chance of making that relationship work. We want you to start thinking, talking and changing. Don't be afraid of the Internet. Include it in your life but, whatever you do, don't let it become your life.

You might be curious about the Internet, worried about your children or partner on the Net, or think you might be addicted to some aspect of it. Whatever your reasons for reading *Online and Personal*, we hope we answer some of your questions and set you on the right path.

Jo Lamble and Sue Morris

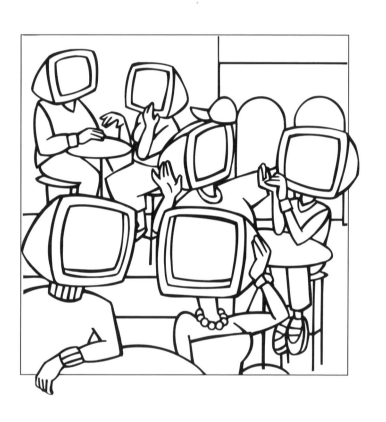

1 The Internet – the good, the bad and the ugly

Kathryn: You'll never guess what? Debbie has left Tim for some guy she's met on the Internet.

Fiona: You're kidding? When? How?

Kathryn: She's apparently been chatting to this guy for six months and no-one knew. She just dropped the bombshell last week that she was leaving.

Fiona: Wow! I'd never have thought she'd be the type to even look at another man.

Kathryn: Me, too. I feel really sorry for Tim, and I wonder what will happen with the kids, as she's apparently going to Canada.

Fiona: I'm totally dumbfounded. This Internet stuff is really scary. My kids are online everyday, and even Bill uses it most nights after work. I have absolutely no idea what they're doing.

Kathryn: Me either. How would you know?

▪ ▪ ▪

We hear so many stories about how someone's life has been affected by the Internet. Some of you may be very familiar with the Internet and its uses; some of you may hope never to have anything to do with it. The rest of you may know the Internet in name only, and not have a clue about what it is or what it does. Kathryn and Fiona's conversation is not uncommon. They are shocked to learn of their friend who is leaving her relationship for a man she's met on the Internet. What's equally worrying, however, is that these women know nothing about the Internet yet their children and partners are regularly online.

In *Online and Personal*, we look at the impact the Internet is having on people's lives. Whether your life has been affected in some way by the Internet or not, we think it is really important to be informed so that you can put in place the necessary safeguards to protect yourself, your children and your relationships. In particular, we want to provide you with strategies that can help you maintain a sense of control in your own life. Let's begin with some of what we do know about the Internet, even though what we do know is changing daily.

The story so far

The Internet is an enormous computer network connecting millions of computers and their users around the world. It's a fabulous communication tool that is changing and will keep changing how we think, interact with people and do business.

Since the Internet (or 'the Net', as it is often called) exploded into our lives it has grown so rapidly that its evolution has out-paced the development of the guidelines that dictate how we 'should' behave within the Internet world. Computer experts, lawyers and psychologists are all struggling to keep up with the development of the Internet. The legal, moral and ethical guidelines are constantly evolving as new situations arise, and so is our understanding of the effects the Internet is having on people and their relationships. Given it's relatively new, we are all learning by trial and error. The good news for those of you who are just starting out with the Net is that you can learn from the experience to date and take action. You can be faster at implementing the safeguards to protect your children and yourself from online problems. We think it is important to understand upfront that the Internet itself is not bad, nor are the problems it presents completely new. Unfortunately, though, it is open to abuse. In the end, it all comes back to how people use the Internet and how they regulate their own behaviour, which is particularly important when you consider how easily the Net infiltrates our lives. There will always be a good, a bad and an ugly side to life, and the Internet is no different.

Let's start with the good.

The good ...

The upside of the Internet is definitely its ability to connect people and businesses all around the world. It promotes the exchange of information, which can benefit business, education and personal relationships alike. For the consumer, you can buy just about whatever you want from wherever you like by shopping online. Similarly, the Internet makes it much easier to access information on any subject. The benefits to education and learning are enormous for both children and adults, and it also is a great form of entertainment.

One of the most distinct advantages of the Net is that it helps us keep in touch with friends and family. It's a great way of maintaining regular contact with friends and loved ones who live in another State or country or travel for work. It offers an easy way to link children to a parent who lives in a different house for example, or children to their grandparents who may live some distance away. Web cams are cameras that can transmit live images over the Internet – they take online communication one step further. Difficult but necessary contact between people, such as ex-spouses who need to communicate with each other about their children, can also be made much easier by way of the Internet.

N E W S F L A S H

A US judge recently ordered a father who had won custody of his 10-year-old daughter to buy himself and the girl's mother computers to allow a video-conferencing system to be set up. The idea was that the mother and daughter could maintain 'live' contact. The court ordered that the mother should have unlimited access to her daughter via the computer – something the father found difficult to accept.

The Sydney Morning Herald 13/2/01

Another plus is that the Internet helps connect people who share similar interests or problems who otherwise would never have easily met. Whether via chat rooms or bulletin boards and the like, the Internet provides an opportunity to get people together from all over the world. Also, as a result of meeting people online, some will go on to have a very happy and normal everyday relationship. If you're in this situation, we suggest a number of strategies in Chapter 3 about how to proceed if you do happen to meet someone via the Net.

The Internet also facilitates communication and promotes a sense of belonging for people who might otherwise be isolated – geographically or because they are elderly, disabled or sick.

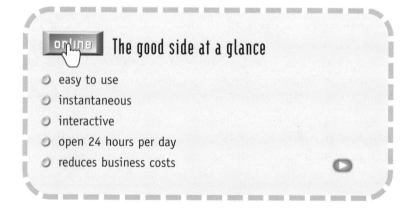

online The good side at a glance

- easy to use
- instantaneous
- interactive
- open 24 hours per day
- reduces business costs

- facilitates international business interactions
- a source of valuable and obscure information
- a form of recreation and entertainment
- helps people stay in touch
- promotes family communication, e.g. children and parents living apart, between grandparents and grandchildren, between adult siblings
- facilitates 'difficult' relationships, e.g. between ex-spouses
- connects people who otherwise wouldn't have met
- facilitates communication when physical access is not easy, e.g. between lecturers and students, for shift workers
- decreases isolation for certain groups of people

N E W S F L A S H

Patients can now email their physical complaints to a doctor's consulting service and receive a written response from a GP or specialist for a fee of A$15.

The Sun Herald 12/00

All in all, the Internet has the power to bring everyone closer together, which has to be good.

The bad ...

We use the umbrella term 'the bad' to refer to those areas where Internet use does not constitute a crime but if left unmonitored or unchecked, the consequences can be damaging to both the user and their relationships. There are four main areas where we can already see the damage: in the workplace; within relationships; children and teenagers; and people who believe they have a problem with their Internet use.

In the workplace

Email is an obvious benefit of the Internet in the workplace. Unfortunately, as with many benefits there is often a downside. Some potential problems include a decrease in face-to-face contact between co-workers, messages being misinterpreted because of the absence of tone and body language, and reduced productivity caused by having to deal with so many emails – especially junk mail and jokes. More serious is the flow of pornographic material between workmates, from the odd crude joke through to hardcore pornographic images. Many people take offence to such material being sent to their computer. Even if they don't receive the material, they may inadvertently view the images on someone else's computer. It can be a form of sexual harassment, and there are likely to be more and more cases of employees being suspended or sacked for sending or viewing such material. We believe that another growing problem in the workplace is Internet abuse by employees who use the Net in work time for their own private purposes.

N E W S F L A S H

Hackers are increasingly using their skills to hack into companies' databases so that they can flood the names on the lists with unsolicited emails.

USA Today 27/9/00

Personal relationships

All types of relationships can be affected by the Net because it can depersonalise communication. It offers an easy route for people to bypass many of the 'niceties' of social interaction. We don't have to look far to see for ourselves. In the name of efficiency many people opt to send email greeting cards or send a quick email instead of making a telephone call. While there are arguments for and against these types of exchanges, the efficiency of the Internet, which is a definite advantage in business, can ironically end up being a huge disadvantage in personal relationships. For some of you these exchanges won't be a problem, but for others they may be hurtful or offensive. Certainly we have heard *I'd rather they didn't send the email thanking me if they could not have been bothered to pick up the phone*. No doubt the next generation won't have the same issues because they'll have grown up with the Internet. We don't think too many people today would send an electronic sympathy card, for example, but it may be an acceptable practice in a few years' time.

You can also get into trouble with your communication on the Net if you respond without giving much thought to what you say. With a click of a button, an email is sent. If harsh words are used, for example, you have to live with the consequences. Recently, we heard of a woman who sent her partner a sexy email thanking him for a wonderful night of passion they had shared. Her partner, obviously feeling quite pleased with himself, forwarded the email on to five of his friends. It's not hard to imagine how devastated the woman was when she found out. The story could have been worse: those five friends could have forwarded the email on to five of their friends and so on. So the motto of the story is: think before you put anything in an email – the consequences can be very far-reaching.

In committed relationships problems can arise if one of you starts getting close to someone else on the Net. Similarly, tension might develop if one of you is doing something on the Net that upsets the other. Examples here include viewing or downloading adult pornography, playing interactive games, compulsive web surfing or working excessively from home. Such behaviour can cause conflict in previously happy relationships.

Single people who are **only** pursuing Internet relationships can also get into trouble. Meeting people only on the Net can sometimes be a real problem because initially you don't really know the person with whom you're communicating. You can't be sure when they're lying and when they're telling the truth. This problem of being uncertain about the truth of the written word is not new. The French dramatist Edmond Rostand wrote the play Cyrano de Bergerac in 1897, based on a seventeenth-century soldier and poet who was disfigured by his grotesque nose. In order to get the lady of his affections to fall in love with him, he wrote the words for another man to say. The question was asked – with whom was the lady falling in love, the man who delivered the words or the man who wrote them? The Internet allows people to pose as whoever they want to be. As long as the relationship takes place solely online, doubt will always exist as to the truth of the written word.

If the relationship progresses, geographical location and finances play a huge part in whether or not you actually meet in person. The danger is that if you can't meet early on, you may end up wasting a lot of time in a relationship that never had a future. You may also have missed out on the opportunity to meet people where you live.

Children and teenagers online

Problems with children and teenagers on the Net include inappropriate online behaviour and excessive Internet contact. Teenagers need to be clear about the rules of acceptable online behaviour, which in a nutshell are no different to the rules of real living. Unfortunately, if a young person's use of the Internet is not well balanced with other important activities, their social and educational development may be jeopardised. Children need to interact face to face with people to develop the social skills required to get on in life – to be assertive, to manage difficult situations, to control their own behaviour and to work with groups of people.

Unfortunately, the Internet can offer an out to children who find social situations difficult. In that way they never learn to face their fears or learn the skills necessary to deal with everyday life. Similarly, if teenagers spend too much time on the Net doing whatever they like, they can't possibly be concentrating on their studies. We think many parents may not realise the full impact of the Internet on their children. Some of you may be comforted by the fact that your children are in front of a computer screen in your own home. While there's some truth in this, you have to ask yourself two questions: *What **are** they doing when they are online?* And, equally important, *What **aren't** they doing when they are online?*

Today's teenagers tend to know more about the Internet than their parents. We call this the ***technological generation gap***. The accessibility of the Internet means that children are being exposed to many more things than we ever could have imagined – or would have allowed into our homes – and so the world is becoming their peer group. To help children resist global peer pressure and keep them on track in their studies and social development, parents need to be informed about the positives and negatives of the Internet, and to work with their children to develop reasonable and safe guidelines.

Internet 'addiction'

Some researchers into the impact of the Internet on people's lives are finding a number of strong similarities between compulsive gambling and Internet addiction, where some estimates suggest that approximately 6 percent of Internet users are addicted. While you might think 6 percent is relatively small, when you actually consider how many millions of people are online worldwide, the numbers are frightening. More significantly, the behaviour of every 'Internet addict' is likely to have a direct effect on at least two, three or four other people. Potentially then, the implications are enormous.

Generally speaking, being 'addicted' means needing more and more of something to get the same positive effect from it. The 'it' as far as the Net is concerned includes: excessive chatting in chat rooms (cyber places where several people can join in conversation with each other); playing interactive games; gambling online; compulsive online shopping; viewing, trading or downloading pornography; and participating in cyber sex and fantasy with people online. (Cyber sex means communicating in a suggestive or erotic manner via the Internet while self-stimulating.) But whatever the activity, when someone feels hooked, they feel out of control. The potential impact on their life is enormous, but they just can't stop.

The bad side at a glance

- has no global 'acceptable use' guidelines
- the written word is open to misinterpretation
- brings offensive pornographic material into the workplace
- decrease in workplace productivity due to excessive personal Internet use
- Internet exchanges are often instantaneous, which precludes a cooling-off period in heated situations
- information on the Net may be inaccurate
- threatens committed relationships by meeting someone else online
- threatens committed relationships by partaking in an activity online that causes conflict with a partner
- difficulties for single people meeting others online – who are they meeting? Will they ever meet face to face?
- teenagers fail to follow the rules of 'real' life online
- teenagers neglect their studies
- it is more difficult to regulate what information your children can access online
- contributes to a loss of social skills
- allows avoidance of real-life social situations/interactions
- is time away from family and friends
- allows neglect of other responsibilities
- it is hard for some people to set their own limits of use
- users may be emotionally and physically unavailable
- online gambling
- compulsive online shopping
- excessive use of pornography/adult websites in the home

As with everything, sometimes it will be hard to distinguish where 'bad' turns into 'ugly'.

The ugly ...

We use the term 'the ugly' to refer to use of the Internet that constitutes a crime, potential crime or an action that most people would consider antisocial. The list includes unregulated access by predators or perpetrators of any kind, including paedophiles, cyber criminals and people hell bent on destroying someone else because of their race, religious beliefs or some other characteristic. Paedophiles are people who feel sexually attracted to children and often seek opportunities to act on their urges; the typical paedophile is an adult in a position of authority with children. The Internet presents a new avenue for paedophiles to prey on unsuspecting children who believe they are safe in their own homes. A child has no idea to whom they are talking, and can unwittingly give out personal details.

N E W S F L A S H

Cyber criminals are finding new ways to perpetrate familiar frauds. Fake investment schemes and auctions without anything to sell are increasing daily.

The Sun Herald 2/01

Similarly, cyber crime is on the increase. Cyber crime targets the computer networks of other people, companies or organisations, and includes hacking into computer systems to 'steal' information, selling information without the user's consent, shutting down major systems just for fun, and being involved with illegal online activities such as child pornography. Cyber criminals work from their computer and are hard to track down.

The increase in 'hate sites', especially in the US, is particularly worrying. A hate site is a website set up to air certain racial or religious prejudices that most people would find intolerable, often in an attempt to recruit vulnerable people. Unfortunately, the anonymity of the Internet provides the perfect breeding ground for hatred because the people who perpetuate it can hide

N E W S F L A S H

A recent Australian conference called 'Cyberhate: Bigotry and Prejudice' was told that hatred and bigotry are increasing on the Internet. The delegates heard that the Net has allowed many peddlers of hate to spread their vicious messages more widely than ever before.

The Sydney Morning Herald 6/11/00

behind their computer screens. It is impossible to tell by glancing at a web page who exactly is behind the site – it may only be one or two individuals who present themselves as a much larger group. The danger lies in whether the people viewing the hate sites are equipped to discern the accuracy or appropriateness of the information. Without regulation, hate sites are a huge problem not easily solved. Similarly, the Internet allows harassment to occur on a much larger scale. Unfortunately, teenagers who were once bullied in the playground can now be the subject of hateful web pages designed by their fellow students. Obviously such behaviour constitutes harassment and needs to be dealt with via the appropriate channels.

 The ugly side at a glance

- child pornography
- hate sites
- cult-like sites
- cyber crime
- sexual assault
- harassment
- stalking
- murder following an Internet association

As we've said, the ugly side of life existed long before the introduction of the Internet. What the Internet offers, however, is a completely new medium for criminals of all types to exploit.

Online and Personal is designed to help people understand the impact of the Internet on their lives and the lives of their children. Whether you personally use the Internet or not, we believe you need to become informed about it. If you think that you or someone close to you might have a problem with Internet use, you need to take action. Many sections of this book will apply to everyone, and others will only apply to some of you. The main aims of this book, therefore, are to:

- help you understand the possible impact of the Internet on your life
- provide basic advice on how to manage the impact of the Internet on your life
- help you educate your children about the Internet
- help you cope if your relationship has been affected by an Internet affair or excessive Internet use
- offer guidelines for meeting people online
- help you break the cycle of excessive Internet use

Let's start with our conclusions

We like to give our conclusions up front so you can keep them in mind as you read through the book. We have developed these conclusions from our work with individuals and couples, and from people who agreed to be interviewed, or contacted us about their stories.

There are five important conclusions we want you to keep in mind:

1. The Internet itself is not the problem – it's how some people use it.
2. Take your time approaching anyone or anything online.
3. Know when to get offline.
4. Internet affairs *are* affairs.
5. Get informed and take action.

Let's look at these conclusions in a little more detail before we take a closer look at who is getting into trouble on the Internet.

The Internet itself is not the problem – it's how some people use it

The Internet readily connects people by decreasing isolation, improving efficiency and facilitating the rapid exchange of information – and like it or not it's here to stay. The types of problems the Net has brought into our lives are not all that different from those we have always faced. What is different, however, is how easily the Net infiltrates our homes. So no matter what limits are set by the powers that be, there will always be some people whose behaviour tests those limits and even exceeds them. Of them, some will feel helpless to control what they do and some will choose to behave in a way that hurts others.

Take your time approaching anyone or anything online

We believe the best way to approach the Internet is by taking your time. The novelty factor will eventually wear off, but in some instances the damage may already be done before this happens. Whether you're surfing the Net, chatting, playing interactive games or visiting adult websites, the aim is to avoid getting into trouble at all costs. Trouble may include: finding yourself involved in some way with a person who does not have your best interests at heart; making a hasty decision about committing to someone you meet online, or becoming hooked on an aspect of the Internet.

Taking your time is particularly relevant to those who may be keen to meet someone online. We know that Internet relationships develop very quickly and people soon believe they know each other intimately. Unfortunately, in Internet relationships you don't have the opportunity to 'test drive' your relationship in the real world nor see your partner's warts. If decisions are made when you're still caught in the bubble of new love, there is a good chance you may regret those decisions. We strongly advise people in Internet relationships to bring their relationship into the 'real world' as soon as possible. If it's not possible, don't pursue the relationship.

Even though the Internet may be the most exciting thing you've been involved with for years, don't fall into the trap of neglecting the rest of your life. By and large it is an exclusive activity, and if you're on the Net you're missing out on other opportunities and invitations.

Know when to get offline

If the estimates that six people out of every hundred are addicted to the Internet are correct, you need to know the warning signs if you use the Internet regularly. If you've tried to cut down your Internet use without success, you may have a problem. Similarly, if someone close to you has complained about your use of the Internet, you may have a problem. We'll discuss the warning signs and offer suggestions for helping you manage your Internet use. We have included our self-help program for you to follow on your own or with your psychologist. The key, however, is admitting that you have a problem. If you don't think you've got a problem then we can't help you.

If you are worried about your partner or your children on the Net, you may find our guidelines useful in helping you gain a greater sense of control over the impact of the Internet on your life.

Internet affairs *are* affairs

If you are in a committed relationship and having an online relationship, you are having an affair. Internet affairs are no different from conventional ones even though some of you may disagree. Affairs are about lies, betrayal, deceit, rejection and lack of commitment. That actual sex has not yet occurred and may never occur in Internet relationships is irrelevant – there is still deceit. Any relationship or 'contact' with another person that removes you or part of you from the relationship with your partner is dangerous.

We'll look at the development of an Internet relationship and how that differs from a conventional one. We'll also offer suggestions of what you need to do if you're involved with someone on the Net, or if your partner is having an Internet affair.

Get informed and take action

We believe that every one of you needs to get informed about the Internet and take action. Whether you are an employer, a partner, teacher, friend, parent or grandparent, someone in your world is involved with the Internet. Don't expect anyone else to put in place the necessary safeguards to protect those you care about, including yourself. You personally need to take action now. Failing to do so will be a mistake. At the end of the day, only if we all work together as a team can we make the Internet a safer place. Ask yourself: *Who has to hear my concerns about the Internet?* It might be your friends, your partner or your government. But if you have children, one thing is for sure: they definitely need to hear your voice. Throughout *Online and Personal* we offer you ideas about how you can become informed about the Internet, regardless of who you are and what your life entails.

What are your concerns?

Now that we have given you our conclusions and highlighted some potential trouble spots, it is worth stopping to assess your concerns about the Internet. Keep in mind your concerns or reasons for reading this book as you go through each chapter.

 My reasons for reading *Online and Personal*

Read through the following list and mentally tick your main reasons for reading a book about the Internet.

- general interest
- education/study
- worried about my children on the Net: amount of time on the Net; activities they partake in; who they are meeting; what they're neglecting; effect on their psychological health

- worried about my partner on the Net with regard to the issues above
- worried about myself on the Net with regard to the issues above
- learning how to prevent problems from occurring: for my children; for my relationship; for myself

The areas you mentally ticked on this list are good indications of where you should focus your attention. We offer many strategies for the different types of Internet issues or problems that we are hearing more about each day. If you are already doing what we advise, keep it up. If not, now is a good time to start.

In brief...

- The Internet easily connects people and businesses around the world.
- Internet addiction is a new problem that will affect people's personal and work life.
- The Internet itself is not the problem – it's how some people use it.
- Take your time approaching anyone or anything online.
- Know when to get offline.
- Internet affairs *are* affairs.
- Get informed and take action.

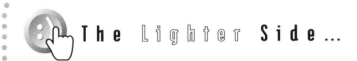

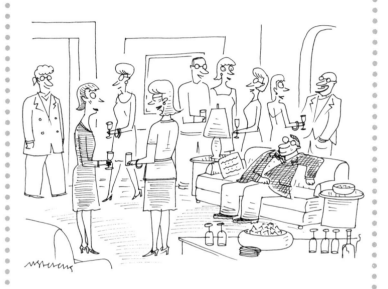

"He's not very exciting in social situations
but on the Net he's a wildman."

‹2› The difference between conventional and Internet relationships

Even though you've all got specific reasons for wanting to know more about the Internet, we guess many of you are interested to learn about the effect the Internet is having on relationships, both the positives and the negatives. Throughout the next few chapters we'll examine how the Internet is changing our relationships. We'll look at how it is becoming the newest dating service for single people, and the effect it is having on existing relationships. And we'll offer some common-sense guidelines to help keep you on track. Now, we want to look at conventional relationships and how they differ from what we know about Internet relationships.

Conventional relationships

Most of you would have had a conventional relationship, and it is worthwhile looking at how such relationships began and matured. When reading through this section, try to think back to a recent relationship you have had or are currently in.

A new relationship

The 'falling' part of falling in love is a pretty amazing experience. Nothing can beat it. In the early days of a new romance, all you can do is think about the other person – where they are, what they are doing, and when you will see them next. There is an urgency to be with them and the intensity is often overwhelming, usually to the exclusion of everything else in your life. As outlined in *Side by Side*, we refer to the initial stage of falling in love as 'the bubble stage'. When two people fall in love it's as if they have been captured in a bubble, floating aimlessly through space and time. How long this stage lasts will be different for each and every one of you.

The bubble

Within the bubble of new love you find a number of important components that all serve to protect the development of the new relationship from outside influences. Perhaps the most well-known component of the bubble is chemistry. It is a mixture of physical and sexual attraction between two people.

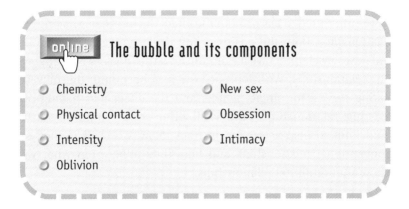

online The bubble and its components

- Chemistry
- New sex
- Physical contact
- Obsession
- Intensity
- Intimacy
- Oblivion

However, the bubble eventually bursts, which is a good thing. But in the beginning a relationship needs its bubble to protect it from outside influences, such as criticism from others, in much the same way that an eggshell protects a growing chick. When the bubble pops, as it always does, you may find out all sorts of things about your partner and their past from which you were being protected. Up until this point you have been somewhat blinded to your partner's warts. Eventually you will see the warts very clearly, as they will see yours. Some warts you will be able to live with, others you won't be able to tolerate. That's why we are such strong advocates of pre-marital counselling. It's far better for everyone concerned if you can find out ahead of time about any major warts that will eventually drive you apart. We actually suggest that couples do not make major decisions, for example, about marriage or parenthood, while they are still floating in their bubble. As you read on, you will see that this is a very important point to remember as far as Internet relationships go.

Intensity and success

Some people fall into the trap of believing that the intensity of the bubble is a good predictor of the long-term success of a relationship. On the contrary, we believe that you have a better chance of enjoying a successful relationship if you allow your relationship to develop slowly. By all means enjoy the bubble phase but don't allow yourself to be blinded by your feelings during this time. It is far better to make a decision about committing to someone based on the facts or evidence. If you make a decision based on your feelings, you may regret it when not only do your feelings change (as they inevitably do), but you uncover your partner's warts. That's why it is necessary to test-drive your relationship in the real world, in the routine of daily life that includes work pressures, illness, competing family commitments and time apart.

Only after the bubble bursts are you in the best position to make a commitment if that's what you choose to do. From then on, if you and your partner do decide to commit to each other, you can work on developing and nurturing a mature relationship that includes love, respect, and lots of hard work.

As you experience different events in your lives, your relationship will naturally be affected by whatever is going on for you – it may be the birth of a child or financial problems. How you and your partner manage the changes you face will determine the success of your relationship. There will always be ups and downs, so keep your expectations realistic. It is important to remember that the perfect relationship does not exist because no-one is a saint or an angel. But what keeps people on the same path together despite their warts is their commitment to each other.

What is commitment?

When most people get married they think they have some sense of what commitment means, especially on their wedding day or the day they decide to move in together. But unfortunately some of this 'sense' gets lost along the way. We believe commitment cannot be understated. We define it as a mindset or a way of thinking that gets played out in everyday life. It goes something like this: *You are the person I choose. No matter what difficulties we face, either as a couple or as individuals, I will be there for you. My behaviour will reflect the fact that I have chosen to be in a relationship with you for the rest of my life.*

Commitment, therefore, is the first step on the path to a successful relationship. Without commitment, a relationship is doomed because there is no incentive to try and solve problems that inevitably arise in all relationships. Commitment is either black or white; there are no shades of grey. Either you are committed to your partner or you're not. It's that simple. If you are already in a committed relationship then you can see from our definition that being stuck in a rut is no excuse to leave a relationship or seek attention elsewhere.

Many people ask us: *What does commitment entail?* To that question we answer that commitment means taking on the responsibility to do whatever is necessary to make your relationship work. That may mean letting go of something you know your partner doesn't like or want, or doing something that is important to them. Commitment also allows you to develop tolerance of your partner's warts. If you are committed to your partner you will be more likely to take the good with the bad. If not, you can always be tempted to bail out.

We see a lot of people who think the grass is greener in someone else's backyard. Unfortunately, the Internet provides access to many more backyards than you could ever have imagined. If you think the grass may be greener elsewhere, you may entertain ideas of divorce if things don't work out. Allowing yourself to think this way undermines commitment. Whenever couples are faced with problems they often ask: *Should we stay together?* We believe that, once you are in a committed relationship, the question instead should become: *How can we make our relationship work?*

When to make a commitment

Since there is no perfect match for anyone, knowing when to make a commitment is an important decision for all couples. Unfortunately, many people don't pay enough attention to how they choose a partner. They often get caught up in how good it feels being together rather than ticking off the factors that in the long run will give the relationship its best chance of success. The factors listed below can help people make a decision about commitment.

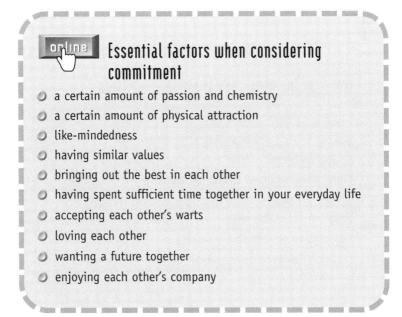

online **Essential factors when considering commitment**

○ a certain amount of passion and chemistry
○ a certain amount of physical attraction
○ like-mindedness
○ having similar values
○ bringing out the best in each other
○ having spent sufficient time together in your everyday life
○ accepting each other's warts
○ loving each other
○ wanting a future together
○ enjoying each other's company

When people have enough of these factors then choosing to commit to the relationship is the next step. Once the commitment is made, the incentive to work on problems as they arise is in place. If the decision made is an informed one, there is less chance of regret.

When not to make a commitment

One simple motto to follow in the beginning is 'If in doubt, don't'. Even if you are worried about hurting someone, or losing someone, it is far better not to commit if you have doubts. We are not suggesting you should end a relationship if you have any doubts about it. Rather we are saying that you should not rush into a commitment before any warning signs have been thoroughly investigated. Warning signs include excessive jealousy, dependency, a controlling nature or indecisiveness.

Is there a commitment problem in your relationship?

There will always be signs of not being committed. These include: flirting with someone else, keeping major secrets from your partner and having an affair. The following list of signs is a good indicator of potential trouble spots.

 The signs of not being committed

- wanting to have a break from the relationship
- making threats about ending the relationship
- having an affair
- not making an effort in the relationship
- ambivalence about life goals (e.g. starting a family, financial commitment)
- keeping the relationship a secret
- pursuing someone else, even if there is no sex involved

- wanting the relationship only on certain terms
- flirting with someone else
- keeping major secrets from a partner
- communicating intimately with someone else on the Internet

Communicating intimately with someone else on the Internet threatens your existing relationship. Many people ask us, *Why?* Often their comments include: *At least we're not having sex; She doesn't care – it's just a bit of fun; It doesn't mean anything.* We totally disagree because when you are getting close to someone on the Net, you cannot possibly be putting the effort into your own relationship that is required to stay on your relationship path.

Internet relationships

We will now compare conventional relationships with Internet relationships. When you start chatting on the Internet you often don't know where your adventure will lead. Your reasons for finding an Internet friend may range from loneliness to curiosity, or you simply might be keen to find the equivalent of a conventional pen friend.

So intimate, so fast

Internet relationships tend to develop very quickly because people report feeling more at ease on the Net than in face-to-face encounters and, as a result, exchange personal information at a much faster rate than in conventional relationships. On the Net there is a tendency to speak on a very intimate level straightaway, and continue to communicate in this way. You can reveal your inner most thoughts and feelings to your online partner. People often say that they thought they had found their soul mate online, because they had never been able to communicate so intimately with anyone before.

The Internet keeps you in the bubble

So what's happening in an Internet relationship? If you think back to the bubble of new love, hopefully you can see how having an intimate relationship on the Internet keeps you in the bubble. All the components of the bubble of new love in a conventional relationship – chemistry, intensity, oblivion, new sex, obsession – are present in an online relationship, except physical contact. Similarly, there is no pressure from the outside world, no time constraints and no avenue for uncovering your e-partner's warts. There is just you and your belief in this perfect partner – your saint or angel, available and understanding. In Internet relationships the couple tend to stay in the bubble because the relationship cannot be incorporated into everyday life – it only occurs on the computer screen and in your heart and mind. Friends cannot meet your partner; family members cannot embrace them into the fold; the relationship cannot be tested under the pressures of work and social life. It's as if the whole world is on hold when you are with your e-partner. This sounds romantic, but it is not realistic.

There's no opportunity for the bubble to burst because this can only happen in the normal chaos of daily living. It is impossible to test-drive an Internet relationship via the computer. If you think about it, there really is not a lot of difference between an e-relationship and a holiday romance. We think most of you would advise a friend not to commit to someone they met while on holidays. An Internet relationship can in fact be more dangerous than a holiday romance because at least on holiday you see them in the flesh. So when someone wants to move overseas to be with their online partner, we'd strongly advise them not to because they are making a major decision while in the bubble of new love, which for any relationship may have diabolical consequences.

What's missing in Internet relationships?

The following chart compares the stages of an Internet relationship and a conventional one. You can see that the bubble stage in an Internet relationship is similar to that of a conventional relationship. One obvious factor that's missing is face-to-face and physical contact. Nothing beats eye contact – that intensive stare, that suggestive look. Cameras linked to your computer may be a starting point, but you are still staring at a camera not into someone else's eyes. Touch, let alone a caress, cannot be achieved on the Internet and it's hard to imagine a relationship without touch. For that matter, all types of body language are important when getting to know someone. Are they affectionate? Are they stand-offish? Do they appear aggressive? Language doesn't give us all the answers to these questions.

Stages of conventional and Internet relationships

	1. The bubble	2. Commitment	3. Mature phase
C O N V E N T I O N A L	Chemistry (offline) Physical contact New sex Intimacy Intensity Oblivion Obsession	Passion & chemistry Physical attraction Bring out the best in each other Time together Accepting each other's warts Enjoying each other's company Loving each other Wanting a future together Like-mindedness Similar values	Managing life changes • children • finances • aging parents • retirement • illness
I N T E R N E T	Chemistry (Online) New cyber sex Intimacy Intensity Oblivion Obsession	Loving each other Wanting a future together Like-mindedness Similar values	

If you look back at our list of essential factors to consider before making a commitment, you will see that two important factors are missing – time spent in everyday life, and acceptance of each other's warts. Neither factor can be assessed in Internet relationships. There are no real-life pressures from work, family or friends. If you have not spent enough (or any!) time in real life you cannot accept each other's warts. If you are not aware of your partner's warts *you cannot make an informed decision to commit.* If you can't make an informed decision, you are setting yourself up for failure and heartache. Internet relationships are a variation of the bubble stage of a conventional relationship, and being aware of this is good news as you can now look to what you need to do if you want to pursue your relationship with your Internet partner.

We now want to spend some time looking at how you can maximise the chance of choosing well if you're single and meeting people on the Net. Then we will look at the effect the Internet is having on committed relationships.

In brief...

- Don't make a commitment to someone while you are in the bubble of new love.
- Internet relationships tend to be very intense from the beginning.
- The Internet keeps you in the bubble.
- If you're unaware of your partner's warts, you can't make an informed decision about commitment.

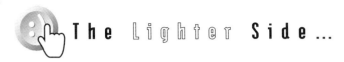

The Lighter Side ...

Gender association

An English teacher was explaining to his students the concept of gender association in the English language. He noted how hurricanes at one time were given only female names, and how ships and planes were usually referred to as 'she.' One of the students raised her hand and asked, 'What gender is a computer?'

The teacher wasn't certain. So he divided the class into two groups: males in one, females in the other, and asked them to decide if a computer should be masculine or feminine. Both groups were asked to give four reasons for their recommendations.

The group of women concluded that computers should be referred to as masculine because:

1. In order to get their attention, you have to turn them on.

2. They have a lot of data but are still clueless.

3. They are supposed to help you solve your problems, but half the time they are the problem.

4. As soon as you commit to one, you realise that if you had waited a little longer, you could have had a better model.

The men, on the other hand, decided computers should definitely be referred to as feminine because:

1. No-one but their creator understands their internal logic.

2. The native language they use to communicate with other computers is incomprehensible to everyone else.

3. Even your smallest mistakes are stored in long-term memory for later retrieval.

4. As soon as you make a commitment to one, you find yourself spending half your paycheck on accessories for it.

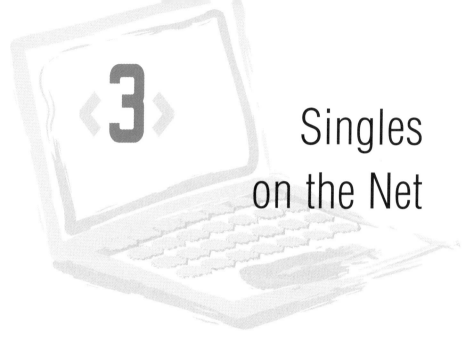

3

Singles on the Net

Many single people complain that they don't know where to go to meet people. Imagine not having to go through the hassle of finding meeting places, searching out those you connect with, before setting about the courting game. It sounds too good to be true, but many people believe chat rooms or Internet dating services offer the perfect solution. In this chapter we highlight the positives and negatives of meeting potential romantic partners on the Net. We offer a number of suggestions that may help you make the best decision if you're using the Net in this way.

The good news first

The Internet is an attractive way to meet people because it bypasses some of the difficulty that often goes along with meeting people in conventional haunts such as pubs, parties, sporting events, adult education courses. Membership of

N E W S F L A S H

Membership of Internet dating services is rapidly on the rise. A recent US newspaper article reported survey results that predicted by the end of 2001, one in five single Americans will use online dating services to find a date.

Meanwhile, Internet dating agencies in Australia have reported staggering increases in membership in the past 6-12 months. Meeting people online is far more common than people previously thought, although many are still reluctant to admit it. One popular service, RSVP, boasts 500 marriages since the site was launched in 1997. Many couples have had to cope with family and friends' scepticism.

The Boston Globe 11/2/01 *and The Sydney Morning Herald,* 31/3/01

Internet dating services is rapidly on the increase. Chat rooms where people who share common interests – music, football or cooking, for example – can talk are popular. Other chat rooms are not interest based, but have a general theme or age range. In this sense, it doesn't seem all that different to attending a course on a specific subject. The big difference is that in a course you may meet say ten to twenty people, whereas on the Net you can potentially meet millions. Being able to meet people this way gives new meaning to the old saying, 'There are plenty of fish in the sea'.

If you do happen to hit it off with someone on the Net, the obvious next step is to meet each other in real life. So in theory it's easy to imagine that such a process can be a real short cut towards friendship or perhaps even an intimate relationship.

When meeting people at a conventional haunt, most people worry about their appearance and their level of social competence and confidence. These kinds of worries can make the idea of going out quite difficult. On the other hand, there are many advantages to meeting people online.

ch@t ─────────➤

Dialogue – Singles		Comments
Anyone?	> hi	
Beeuty	> pleased to meet u I'm m/30/Adelaide	*Beeuty is a 30-year-old male who lives in Adelaide*
Anyone?	> then try betty	*Obviously, someone called Betty would be good for him to chat to*
Beeuty	> rotfl why betty	*rotfl = Rolling on the floor laughing*
Cando	> hiya	
Anyone?	> she loves Adelaide men	
Beeuty	> tnx who do you like	*tnx = thanks*
Anyone?	> I like using a firm grip...lol	*Sexual reference – no restrictions here*
		lol = laugh out loud
Beeuty	> You want to whisper	*whisper = an invitation to have a private chat*
Cando	> What's your sit...married/single/kids/etc	*sit = situation*
Anyone?	> Happily single 1 dog 1 cat	
Cando	> Sounds perfect	
Cando	> I'm married if you can call it that	*Divulging personal problems to strangers*
Anyone?	> Ohh that's no good	*Gets the attention he wants*
Desperado	> Any ladies like to phone me	
Anyone?	> Why don't you just whisper	
Desperado	> It's not working	
Anyone?	> Aww too many give up on marriage nowadays	
Cando	> She didn't get home til 7am the other nite... the guy I was already sus about dropped her off.	*More personal information – true or not?*

Anyone?	> Cheer up ol son	*Anyone? is clearly trying not to be dragged into it*
Farout	> Hello again	
Tanked	> WB Farout How u been	*WB = welcome back*
Farout	> Not bad tnx an u	
Babe2000	> Alo xo)	*Alo xo) = hello kiss, big hug*
Beeuty	> C ya everyone	
Babe2000	> What colour eyes have you got tanked	*Flirtatious remark*
Tanked	> Brown	
Babe2000	> My eyes are chocolate brown	
Tanked	> Mine are just brown	
Babe2000	> Do you have a lovely smile	*And another*
Tanked	> It's OK	
Babe2000	> What are you into	
Tanked	> Movies cycling reading music	
Tanked	> Are you married	
Babe2000	> Maybe	*And another*
Tanked	> Are you engaged	
Babe2000	> No. Are you engaged	
Farout	> She's a flirt	*Fair comment from someone watching this interchange*
Tanked	> No, but I got a really nice friend though	
Babe2000	> Are you married	
Tanked	> No	
Babe2000	> Are you close	
Tanked	> I would like to be in about 12 months	
Farout	> I like watching you flirt	
Babe2000	> Keep watching I'm good	*And another*
Farout	> How good, show me	
Babe2000	> You wish	
Babe2000	> You sound like a nice guy tanked	*Realises Tanked isn't getting into flirting and pays him some respect for it*

Advantages of meeting people on the Net

- it's easy and fun
- it's fast
- there is a novelty factor about meeting someone from a different country
- can be too tired to go out but not to go online
- can be online in pyjamas
- can easily leave a conversation that's going nowhere, without having to make an excuse
- don't have to be worried about your appearance
- can get to know what someone is like without any pressure to have sex
- there's no chance of catching sexually transmitted diseases (STDs)
- can be less anxiety-provoking
- it can be easier to express yourself online
- it can be more time-efficient
- dating services facilitate introductions by using online profiles and photographs
- can meet people who share the same interests
- can meet people through online groups who are experiencing similar problems, e.g. a particular disability or disease
- can meet people at similar life stages, e.g. widowed, retired

Peggy and Julian talk of how they met in a chat room, fell in love, and then met in real life. Their stories offer a good insight into how an Internet romance can flow into lifelong commitment.

▶ Peggy's story [21 years]

When I was seventeen, I was living at home in West Virginia, United States, and was studying at school. I convinced my mother to buy a computer to help me with my schoolwork and my interest in graphic design. My friends had already left school, and so I also wanted to go online to keep in touch with them. Mum baulked at the idea because she was worried about how much it would cost to use the Internet. Mum came around and I went online. The first chat room I visited was set up for fans of the rock band Nine Inch Nails. In the room I made many friends. Some of these friends have also ended up being real-life friends. One even ended up living up the corridor from me in college.

A good friend I met on the Net then set up her own chat room and I went in there. It was there that I met Julian. I had seen him around the room for a while, and we had made a few passing remarks to each other from time to time. We started to get to know each other properly from that August. We were just friends for almost two years. Both of us had some pseudo-relationships online, but they were just shallow infatuations with people. When the relationships would end, we would console each other as friends. We started chatting using voice programs and exchanged photos and gifts. We then started talking on the telephone.

When we eventually got together, we didn't rush into a commitment, we just talked about how we felt and decided it would be good to meet each other and see how it went. One day, Julian just stated that he was coming to the US. He had left school just prior to making this decision, so I worried that he had left school to be with me. I didn't want him to do that, because we had not made any sort of commitment to each other. He reassured me that he had left school because he was unhappy there, not so that he could be with me.

He arrived in the August and as soon as I got over my anxiety (about twenty minutes) we just clicked. I had never been so comfortable with anyone in my life. I trusted him completely. He stayed with me in my flat. I was working, and he hung around. He met my family and friends. I must admit that when he first came over, I had expected the relationship to be perfect. There was a rough patch there for a while as we discovered each other's faults. Commitment taught me how to respect each other despite our faults.

After a while, we started realising that we were serious about each other. He asked me to marry him in October. I said 'yes', even though I didn't know how we would do it. Julian was not going to be able to move over to the States. In November, Julian flew back to Australia. We were engaged, but the next step was a mystery.

I madly started saving money and Julian landed a good job in Sydney. One month after he left, my job fell through and I had to move back home. The stress of being apart was so hard. It was actually much harder to be apart after we had met in real life. We wanted to be together, but we didn't know how. My mum realised how miserable I was and told me to go to Australia. She lent me the money for my ticket. I flew out in April 2000. I had never flown past Ohio before, so I was a bit scared.

When we met again, it was as if an ache had been lifted. We got married on 17 June here in Australia. The day itself was very special, but extremely difficult without my parents. The first few months were tricky as I couldn't work and had no support here. Julian only had limited support too, since his family and friends were in Melbourne.

Now, things are going smoothly. I think the hard part is over. He amazes me. He is my soul mate. If we do have a fight, I think 'We shouldn't be fighting – we have crossed continents to be together'. We are a real team now. My advice to anyone who meets someone on the Net is that if you feel a spark, take the risk. But keep your eyes open. Don't expect fireworks. Be realistic. If it doesn't work out, you can always make a really good friend. ◄

► Julian's story [18 years]

I first went online when I was fifteen years old. I was living in rural Victoria with my parents. We had the Internet connected at home through my mum's work so there were restrictions placed on ▶

its usage. I quickly worked out how to get around these limits and found a great chat room that was based in Singapore. There was no offensive talk, no racism or bigotry, just some nice people getting to know each other. A girl I met in this chat room recommended another cool site that had a music theme to it. A teenager in the States had set it up herself. The restrictions placed on our home Internet use hadn't caught up to this new site and so it was easy to access. It was in this second chat room that I met Peggy.

I had some close relationships with girls on the Net, and made some good friends too. People earn good and bad reputations on the Net. Friends warn you about some people and encourage you to meet and chat to others. I truly believe that with good judgement, there's no danger on the Internet. I certainly gained a lot of confidence going online.

Once Peggy and I got together on the Net, I just wanted to fly over and meet her. I wasn't scared. I knew I had someone I could trust. I loved her. I told my parents the day my passport arrived in the mail. When we met, it was very physical. Sex had not been an issue on the Net, and so we could let go of all our inhibitions online. Meeting in person enabled the relationship to continue, rather than to begin again. We were building on our Internet relationship. Although I must admit that as a seventeen-year-old, I was rather naive about the differences between an online relationship and real life.

I was totally committed to Peggy and wanted to marry her. I didn't like the US and so did not know how we could be together. After I returned home, I moved to Sydney and got a great job. I started paving the way for Peggy to come. When she came, it just seemed to be the right thing to get married, and I know it was. We are now finding our own niche and have started making our life together. Even though we have been together for two years, this will be our first Christmas together. Peggy's family are coming over and they will be having Christmas with my family.

My advice to anyone having a relationship on the Net is to take it slowly. ◀

Like Julian and Peggy, there are of course many people who go on to form wonderful relationships from the Net. If you're in an online relationship, the suggestions we make in **The single person's 'do' list** later in this chapter may help increase the likelihood of success in the future. Because the Internet is so new, it's too early to tell how successful relationships like these will be compared to those that began face to face.

N E W S F L A S H

One recent trend is cyber weddings. Couples can have an intimate ceremony in front of a web cam so that any family members and friends who are not invited can feel part of the event.

The Sun Herald 1/01

Now for the bad news

As you can see, there are lots of advantages to meeting online. We certainly believe that the number of people meeting online will continue to increase over the next few years. But we believe there are definite disadvantages to meeting people online, and some hidden dangers.

The disadvantages

If you meet someone online you run the risk of forming an inaccurate perception of who they are. You need to accept that your initial opinion could be wrong because you only have access to a very limited amount of information. In the end, if you do eventually meet and realise the person isn't who you thought or expected them to be, you've probably wasted a lot of time. In that way, an Internet relationship is quite ironic because often it is the 'easy' side of Internet relating that is attractive in the first place, but in the end the whole process may turn out to be more long-winded than if you had met someone by conventional means.

There are many potential problems with meeting someone online, including misinterpreting what is written, making an inaccurate judgement about someone, losing social skills and confidence, missing out on opportunities to meet someone else, and putting yourself in real danger. Let's take each of these separately.

Misinterpretation of the written word

Remember that communicating only via the written word is fraught with difficulties. Misunderstandings can easily occur and it's difficult to check out the 'neediness' of the person with whom you are communicating, because you are removed from their environment and other sources of important information.

Inaccurate opinions

When we meet and get to know a person we form an opinion about them based on a number of pieces of information we pick up. We get our information from:

- the chemistry that does or doesn't exist
- how they interact with their friends
- how they treat their parents and siblings
- their manners and general behaviour
- and their overall appearance

When we solely rely on the written word we miss out on all this information. Without knowing if there is any physical chemistry between the two of you, it is easy to either tell yourself that physical chemistry is not that important or convince yourself that it will be present when you get together, even if you find that it's not. There can be dire consequences once the real-life relationship is well established because the relationship was built on wishful thinking.

By not seeing someone with their friends, how can you answer the following questions: *Are they a leader or a follower? Are they rude or respectful? Are they a good listener?* Similarly, seeing your partner with their family gives you insight into their values and their sense of entitlement and appreciation.

We learn a lot about people by what we observe of their behaviour, not just what we are told. For example, it is very helpful to see how your partner eats, whether they are well-mannered, how they treat people they meet in everyday life, such as shop assistants and waiters. Also, you want to know whether they drive recklessly, litter, or push their way through a crowd. No matter how much you tell yourself that looks are not important, we do learn a lot about a person from the way they dress, how they walk, and their general appearance.

The loss of social skills

By relying on the written word, it can be easy to slowly lose some of your social skills. It can be easy for example to forget the art of small talk. Knowing the boundaries of conversation and personal space is not important when online. On a computer there are no nonverbal cues such as eye contact or body language to be given or interpreted. No real manners are needed. You do not need to wait your turn or learn how to gradually break into a formed group. By not practising these difficult skills when online, it can be easy to forget how to use them and make it all the more difficult when you find yourself in a face-to-face situation again.

Losing confidence

Without social skill practice, your self-confidence can rapidly decline. Some people may start off socially confident but after a while find themselves avoiding situations as they feel less sure of themselves. There are others who always found social interactions difficult and opt for the Internet because it is not as confronting. With decreasing confidence come anxiety, avoidance and social withdrawal. At this point it becomes hard to meet anyone in person, even if the relationship did begin online.

Missed opportunities

Not everyone who forms an Internet relationship lives close by, let alone in the same country. Spending a lot of time chatting to people on the Net also takes time away from meeting people in real life and developing friendships. If you are getting intimate with one particular person on the Net, there is no incentive to look around for anyone else. If this special person to whom you are chatting turns out to be your future real-life partner, that's great, but if that relationship doesn't make the transition into real life, you have wasted a great deal of time and perhaps missed opportunities to meet someone else.

In real life we would encourage anyone to move on from a relationship that has no future – the same advice applies to Internet relationships. The problem is it can often take a long time to determine whether a Net relationship will stand the test of time. We would advise anyone chatting on the Net to maintain their normal social life as well. Make sure you are getting out with people for at least part of the time.

The dangers

There was an episode of the TV show 'Ally McBeal' that had Ally up on a statutory rape charge for having cyber sex with a minor. A fairly humorous attempt at addressing an ever more relevant issue was made. Ally thought she was having an 'affair' with a man. The teenager knew she was older and thought he could learn from her. In court, Ally was acquitted because the prosecution could not prove she knew he was a minor. If you are single, how do you know the person to whom you are chatting is not a minor, or someone who is needy, has a criminal record or a serious psychological problem? You may end up investing a lot of time in a doomed relationship at the expense of other potentially successful ones. That time cannot be reclaimed, and neither can the confidence in your own judgement and trust in other people you may have lost.

N E W S F L A S H

Police have identified three types of cyber stalking:
1. Threatening emails, viruses, and sending high volumes of junk mail (the most common form).

2. Internet stalking, involving slandering and endangering victims on the Net.
3. Computer stalking, where the perpetrator assumes control over the computer of a targeted victim.

The Sydney Morning Herald 8/1/00

 To whom are you chatting?

In your diary or notebook, describe your Internet partner.

- What do you like about them?
- What would you like to know more about?
- Is there anything so far that concerns you about them or what they have told you?

What do you do now?

Now let's look at what steps you can take to keep yourself safe on the Net. We begin with those of you who might just have started chatting but have not yet connected with anyone in particular.

 The single person's 'do' list

- Go to chat rooms that are clearly for a certain age or interest group.
- Chat to people who live fairly close by.
- If you use an Internet dating service, connect with people who live close by.
- Organise to talk with them at another time to test their sincerity.

- After a while, arrange to meet them face to face in a group, in a public place, and for a limited time.
- Continue to meet other people in real life.

If you are single and perhaps are finding that you are starting to 'speak' to one or two particular e-friends then you need to be sure you continue to protect yourself on the Net. We mean protect yourself physically and emotionally. Our guidelines, listed in the following table, are designed to help you *take your time* when developing relationships with e-partners. You may get to the point that eventually you want to disclose more personal information, but we would warn you not to do this too early. The fact that the communication has been very intimate does not mean you truly know someone.

 The single person´s `don´t´ list

- Don't use your real name.
- Don't give out your email, home or work address.
- Don't send a photo of yourself.
- Avoid anyone who uses language that makes you uncomfortable.
- Don't lie online because eventually you may meet.
- Don't give out your phone number or talk on the phone too early.
- Don't accept invitations to meet anyone alone in private.
- Don't think you know someone just because the communication has been intimate.
- Don't be surprised when someone turns out to be quite different in person.
- Don't stop meeting people in real life.

If you decide that you do want to meet in person, start with a telephone call, followed by a meeting in a public place. If that first meeting goes well, don't assume everything is fine. If you want to meet again, we recommend you do this publicly, too. You still need to follow through with what we call your 'safety check', which we discuss in the next section. If you don't want to see your e-partner again let them know in no uncertain terms that a relationship with them is not for you. Some of you may find this difficult but it is better for both of you to be direct. You also have to be prepared for your e-partner to veto any further contact.

Will you meet your e-partner?

We want to now look at how realistic it is for you to bring your relationship with your e-partner into the real world. We'll suggest what to do if you think you'll never meet and what steps you should take if you think there is a possibility for you to meet.

No chance of meeting

If you can't see a way to meet your e-partner in real life, we suggest you both agree to a 'no-go' period of six months. This buffer allows you to make a break and think more clearly about your situation. Contract with yourself to:

- limit all Internet contact
- increase your real-life activities
- allow yourself time to grieve
- think in a helpful way, e.g.: *It's better to move on now than in twelve months' time*
- avoid at all costs recontacting your Internet partner in that time

If after six months you do recontact each other, you need to re-evaluate whether your situations have altered. If they haven't, you need to make a complete break and work towards rebuilding a life where you live. If you believe your relationship has no future, it's better to call it quits as soon as you can.

If you find yourself still longing to be with your Internet

partner despite there being little chance that you will meet, it may help to ask yourself:

- Do I want to be in this situation in one year's time, or five years' time?
- What do I stand to lose by holding on to this hope that we will be together at some stage?

We find it useful to use the analogy of being interested in someone who is married. A married person is technically not available so there is no point in pursuing them. If your e-partner lives on the other side of the world and it is practically impossible for the two of you to meet, they are not available either. If you do believe you can eventually meet in real life, but not for some time, a 'no-go' period is still not a bad idea as it allows you to re-evaluate your decision based more on fact, not the bubble of new love.

A chance of meeting

If there is a chance you may meet your e-partner, it becomes very necessary to do a safety check on them. You need to find out as soon as possible:

- What is their real name, age and sex?
- Are they married?
- Do they really do what they claim to?
- What is their family background?
- Do they have a criminal record?

Such a check may sound unromantic, but we believe you need to uncover as much information as possible about your e-partner. If you were meeting people through a conventional dating service, you would assume there were some safeguards in place. For example, you would hope the agency had done a criminal check and had looked at personality profiles. When you meet someone online there are no safeguards unless you put them in place yourself. If you do, however, use an Internet dating service, you still need to find out this type of information for yourself.

Unfortunately many people feel embarrassed or guilty about not 'trusting' their new e-partner. But where's the logic in that?

Would you be offended if they checked you out in some way? It is useful to think about the safe sex practices at the beginning of the twenty-first century. Adults see it as normal to ask a prospective sexual partner about their HIV status before entering into a sexual relationship with them. In the early Eighties, however, most found this a difficult question to ask – they thought they didn't have a right to know.

It all comes back to the need to develop a personal 'code of conduct' with regards to Internet behaviour for everyone – single, married, young, old – who uses the Internet. As we keep saying, don't expect anyone else to do it for you. Don't assume that everything someone tells you is true. Don't expect you are always a good judge of character. But if you keep all of this in mind as you develop an Internet relationship, you're off on the right foot.

Before you get to the point of making a long distance or international trip, you need to do some checking. Our hunch is there could be a correlation between distance and lying. That is, the further away a person lives, the more likely you are to lie or be lied to.

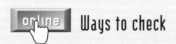 **Ways to check**

- Check their place of work – make a phone call.
- Compare what you've been told in earlier emails with more recent communication – does it add up?
- Access records of births, deaths and marriages.
- Hire a private investigator.

What happens when Internet lovers meet?

If you are having a relationship with someone on the Net, you may like to hear what often happens when Internet lovers meet.

High expectations

Because there has often been a very intensive start to the relationship, the meeting can be very electric. Chemistry that was evident online will often be transformed into traditional physical chemistry. The intensity and high level of intimacy of the online communication often leads people to *expect* instant chemistry and closeness. These expectations can run high. For many, the sparks are there and a new hunger develops for learning everything else there is to know about this person. The bubble of new love continues and it can be a very exciting and fulfilling time. If the instant sparks are not evident, however, the disappointment can be overwhelming. The risk is that you'll suppress your disappointment and try to talk yourself into believing that chemistry does exist, because you so much want it to be there.

▶ Tracey's story (29 years)

My story is one I'm embarrassed about, but as no-one knows my real name, I'll tell it to help others avoid making the same mistake as me.

I suppose you'd say that I've never been lucky with relationships. I would love to be married but the few relationships I've had have never lasted very long. I find it really hard to meet guys I like and feel awkward around them. I end up spending a lot of time at work, on my own or with my married friends who are always trying to set me up with someone or another.

About a year ago or so, I began using chat rooms. In the back of my mind I think I saw it as a safe place to meet people and I found talking via the Internet much easier for me socially. I no longer felt awkward and actually enjoyed meeting people from interesting places. It didn't take long before I met someone special, who I will call Bob. We had lots in common, and I thought I might have met my match. Before long we exchanged photos and started telephoning each other. As we lived on opposite sides of the world, it took us longer to meet than if we lived in the same city or country. We both were very keen to meet so we started planning our first meeting – a vacation together. For lots of reasons it worked out that Bob would travel to meet me.

As our first meeting drew near, it's hard to convey in words how I actually did feel at the time. It all seemed so unreal, standing at the airport waiting for someone I'd never set eyes on in my life before. I felt a tremendous mix of excitement and nervousness. It was as if I was a teenager again going on that first special date when you can't stop shaking and feeling nauseous. But I knew as soon as we hugged, Bob wasn't my perfect match. My heart sank and I felt physically sick. It wasn't going to work. I'd made a mistake; a huge mistake.

I then found myself in a terrible predicament – this guy holding on to me had just flown halfway around the world for a two-week vacation. What did he think? What was he expecting? I can clearly remember feeling the panic rising within me as I considered my options. How was I going to get out of this situation? What if he wanted sex? Would he get angry? Would we still be friends?

Bob sensed my awkwardness and, luckily for me, he handled it pretty well and was a gentleman about it. I ended up spending two days with him before he ventured off on his own. It still gives me shivers down my spine when I think about that time. I feel guilty about the whole thing, but have to remind myself that I didn't do anything wrong. We no longer are in touch – it was all too hard.

Looking back, I think I wanted a relationship so much that I never considered that I might not like him when we actually did meet. It's difficult though, because there's no other way we could have met sooner. My advice to others is to meet up as soon as you can but accept that there is a risk involved – a risk that it might all backfire. ◀

Expectations can be unrealistic when it comes to looks, life context and ongoing communication. You may have sent photos to one another, but no doubt these were the very best you could find. You know that looks are not the most important factor in a relationship, but when you begin a relationship face to face you know exactly how that person looks. When it starts online you cannot help but have expectations about looks, which are probably completely unconscious.

You may have been communicating with your Internet lover for weeks, months or maybe years. You may have heard all about their work, their friends and their family. You will have formed an image about their day-to-day life that becomes part of your expectations about them. These expectations are tested when you actually meet. The work life may not be as glamorous as you had imagined. It may take up more time than you had hoped. Their family may not be as welcoming as you had expected, and their friends may not be as accepting as you had wished. You need to prepare yourself for such views. Their home may not be quite what you had pictured and their taste in clothes, furniture and music may not match your image. The difference between your expectations and reality needs to be digested, and adjustments made to your thinking.

Most common is an unrealistic expectation about communication. Talking online invites such intimacy and self-disclosure because it is deemed to be safe and inhibitions are lowered. Meeting and beginning a relationship face to face creates a new ball game. Inhibitions are raised and self-consciousness returns to some degree and may lead to reduced levels of intimacy and openness. The disappointment that your Internet lover is not using the sort of language they used online can be profound.

As a result of these potential discrepancies between expectations and reality, many people ask themselves: *Who is this person?* or *Is this the same person I fell in love with?* The answer is 'yes', this is the same person but this is the real or whole person you now need to get to know. It might be useful to keep in mind our representation of conventional and Internet relationships that we drew for you in Chapter 2. As you can see, an Internet relationship is similar to the bubble or first phase of a conventional relationship. If you think this way then you have a far better chance of managing the discrepancies between your expectations of your Internet partner and reality.

Think of this meeting as a new beginning. Once you meet your Internet partner and start dating in the true sense of the word, they cease to be your Internet partner. He or she is now *your partner* and you're beginning a *new* relationship. You are now in the bubble stage of a conventional relationship and your relationship has a long way to go. Take your time and get to know each other in all the ways that have not been possible over the Net. Find out what it would be like to hold hands, take a ferry ride, share a meal. Experience the simple things in life. Try to slowly drop your old 'Internet' image of your partner and develop a new one. If you look towards the future without comparing the two images of your partner, you stand a greater chance of beginning a healthy, mature relationship.

In brief...

- There are many advantages to meeting people on the Internet.
- The written word can be misinterpreted.
- It is possible to lose confidence and social skills by restricting your social life to the Internet.
- It is impossible to fully know someone without meeting them.
- If you do meet someone on the Net, take your time.
- Keep your expectations realistic.

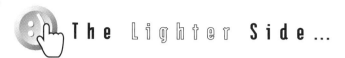

The Lighter Side...

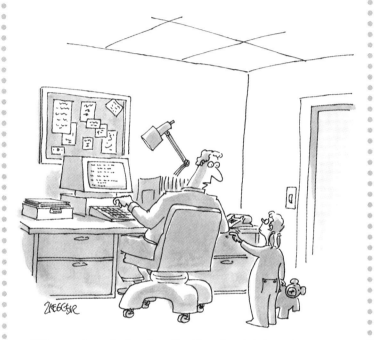

"Honey, please don't talk to Daddy when he's in a chat room."

4

Is the Internet affecting your relationship?

The Internet can be a trap. The defining features of this new technology make it potentially addictive, and like any drug, if abused, the effects on the user and those closest to them can be detrimental. Whether or not you believe your Internet use is affecting your relationship with your partner, it is important for you to be aware of the warning signs that spell potential trouble. Typically it will be the user's partner who first draws attention to the problem because the user is living a life of fantasy on the Net. In this chapter we look at the effect the Internet is having on committed relationships. In the following chapter we suggest what you can do to take control of the situation, whether you're a user or the partner of a user.

The problem for committed relationships

The caller sounded desperate: *Please reassure me that there's nothing wrong. My wife spends most of her day in chat rooms on the Internet. She hardly does anything around the house or with the kids any more – only the bare minimum. When I confronted her about what she's doing, she got angry and told me it was none of my business. I'm at a complete loss because I feel that she's slipping away from me.*

●　●　●

Unfortunately, in our practice we are hearing about more and more people whose existing relationships are being threatened by Internet romances or other Internet activities such as the use of adult websites and interactive games. Where should the line be drawn about what behaviour is acceptable and what is unacceptable or dangerous? There tends to be three groups of people whose behaviour on the Net poses a problem for their committed relationships. First there are those who are curious about the Internet who end up becoming hooked on some activity that takes them away from their committed relationship. It doesn't always have to be another person. Certainly, the use of excessive pornography and interactive games can cause even the best of relationships to become unstuck. The second group includes those who actively seek excitement and novelty on the Internet, or someone else, because they are unhappy in their relationship. The third group is made up of those people who didn't realise something (usually intimacy) was missing in their relationship until they unintentionally met someone else. Instead of working on their real-life relationship, they pursue their Internet lover, believing them to be their saint or angel. Regardless of which group you are in, our suggestions in the next chapter can help you get your relationship back on track.

Curiosity killed the cat

It is important to remember that not everyone who starts chatting on the Net, playing games or surfing the web does so because they are unhappy in their marriage. We believe a number of people begin using the Net because they are curious about what it has to offer. There is a voyeur in all of us. It is fun, exciting and definitely stimulating. But then they can't stop – just one more look; just another hour; just another game. The Internet can be seductive. So our warning is – if your partner is complaining about your Internet activity, don't dismiss their complaints, listen to them. Relationships can easily be neglected and before you know it your relationship is dead. If your partner is often on the Net, speak up as soon as you realise that their online behaviour is worrying you.

Behaving like an ostrich

Some people whose relationships end up in trouble because of the Internet are like ostriches – they avoid facing important issues and problems. Before long ostriches, who possibly have been unhappy for some time but have not spoken up, have turned their attention to someone or something on the Internet. It is now too late for the relationship to be salvaged as the ostrich wants to run away, or their partner wants out.

Something is missing

People who meet someone special on the Net are not always unhappy in their real-life relationship. What happens is that the new Internet relationship offers a level of intimacy that they realise has been missing in their real-life relationship. Instead of turning their attention to how they can improve the level of intimacy, they pursue their Internet lover, believing that they have found 'the one' for them.

N E W S F L A S H

According to a visiting psychologist from the US, Internet addicts fall into three categories: those who go online to escape their real-life problems, those who pretend to be someone else online, and those who indulge in pornography and/or cyber sex.

The Sydney Morning Herald 4/5/01

ch@t

Dialogue

John	> Hi Jill. Please pm me.

Jill > I didn't know if you would come on today. Didn't you say yesterday that you had to go somewhere with your wife?

John > I was meant to, but we had another big fight. It's hopeless trying to talk to her. That's why I like chatting with you so much.

Jill > How long have you been having problems?

John > For years. She is always criticising me. She hasn't got a nice thing to say to me.

Jill > I can't believe that. You sound so wonderful. I can't think of a bad thing to say to you.

John > Yeah, you and I can talk so easily. I feel as if you know me far better than my wife. I wish you lived near me so we could meet.

Jill > What would your wife say about you meeting me?

John > She probably wouldn't care. She knows the marriage is over as well as I do.

Jill > My marriage has been over for years We just stay together for Jesse's sake.

John > You are a wonderful mother. Of course you would think of Jesse first.

Comments

Have obviously spoken before. No longer wants to talk in general chat room. Will start to talk in private. pm = private message

Checking up on his movements with his wife.

Telling a 'stranger' about his marital problems.

She cannot possibly know him well enough to say anything bad (except his lack of commitment to his marriage).

A very common line.

How would he know what sort of a mother she is?

Jill	> I actually think Jesse would be all right if we split up. He could come with me, or even stay with Nick.	*Starting to have irrational thoughts.*
John	> Maybe he should stay with Nick, and you could come over here and be with me.	
Jill	> You don't mean that do you? Would you really leave her for me?	*Asks him for a commitment.*
John	> In a flash – if you say you would come.	*He gives it.*
Jill	> I think I'm in love with you and I haven't even met you.	
John	> I know I love you. You don't have to see someone to know and love them. I loved you after one week of talking talking to you. I could just tell we were soul mates and that we were meant to be together.	*They begin to convince themselves that it's unimportant that they haven't met.*
Jill	> What should we do now? Maybe, I should just pack up and leave soon.	*Willing to give up everything.*
John	> Why don't you come over for a holiday first. You could say that you had a business trip and we could have a week together.	*He sounds a bit worried about committing to her now.*
Jill	> Or you could do the same thing and come here. It would sound more convincing if you had a business trip.	
John	> I have been on too many lately. If you came here, I could show you the most wonderful time. Think about it.	*Not willing to take the risk. Wants her to be the one.*
Jill	> That's all I will think about.	

■ ■ ■

Jill	> Hello my darling. I am online now. Nick is home, so I don't know how long I will be able to talk. But I will try to get back on between 1 and 2 p.m. I miss you terribly. Anyway I better go … Nick might wake up in any minute. Love you very much sweetheart … always and forever.	*Deceiving her husband. Behaviour becoming riskier.*
John	> I'll check back in between 1 and 2, your time. I love you too.	

■ ■ ■

Jill	> I'm back online. Are you there? Did you miss me?	
John	> I miss you all the time. I want you to	*A very intense*

know something I don't do one night stands. I want to be with you. I do not love my wife and she doesn't love me. I haven't made love to her for two years. I am so much in love with you sweetheart. I have never felt this way about anyone in my life. I hope you believe me.

response to the question: Did you miss me?

Jill > I wish I had met you years ago. Then I wouldn't have married Nick and I wouldn't have to go through the hassle of divorce. Where were you then?

John > It doesn't matter where I was. I'm here now – waiting for you.

⬚ ⬚ ⬚

John > I couldn't wait to get up this morning and see if you had emailed me, and you had! I just can't put into words the way I feel about you. I didn't know love could be like this. That's why I get jealous of you talking to the other guys in the rooms. I trust you but I don't trust them. Perhaps if you just sent me your picture it would help me to cope with the emptiness I feel without you. I know all those other guys want your pic too, but they don't have what we have.

All this intimacy and declarations of love, and they haven't even seen a picture of each other.

Jill > I'll send you mine if you send me yours. You were the one who said it didn't matter what we looked like.

John > It still doesn't matter, but it will make it easier to dream about you if I knew exactly what you looked like.

Jill > I'll go and have one of those make-over sessions and send you a really sexy shot.

John > You could send me a photo of you in a sack and I would think it's sexy.

Jill > OK I will. I better go. Nick is coming home early today because we are going over to his mum's for her birthday. Dream of me in my sack.

Still living a married life while having an affair. To whom is she committed?

John > I dream of you every night. Talk to you tomorrow and forever.

Internet relationships are affairs

Many people think Internet relationships are permissible because they don't cross the conventional sexual boundary. We disagree: if you're in a committed relationship and involved with someone on the Net, you are breaking the bond of your commitment to your partner. Maybe you are only chatting about personal details, maybe you're flirting or maybe you're only having 'meaningless' cyber sex. But any relationship or 'contact' with another person that removes you or part of you from the relationship with your partner is dangerous. Gina's story highlights how easily relationships can develop under your nose and before you know it, your partner wants to leave.

 online **Why Internet relationships are affairs**

- because getting close emotionally to someone else risks your relationship and threatens your commitment to your partner
- because communicating intimately takes you away from your relationship
- because deceit is usually involved at some level
- because actual sex is only one dimension of an affair

▶ **Gina's story [39 years]**

Mark and I have been married for twelve years. When our son was three, Mark suffered a serious spinal injury. He was hospitalised for six months. We weren't sure whether he'd live, let alone walk. Nothing prepared me for the nightmare that followed the accident. I was pregnant, I had to sell our house, have our daughter, find a new house, and look after Mark.

After six months, he came home in a wheelchair. Slowly he began to walk again. I had help with the children and with the housework, but I nursed him around the clock. Seven years later, he can now get around, but needs help cooking, cleaning and doing all the little tasks that require coordination. He is still regarded as severely disabled. Sex has been nearly impossible which has been hard on both of us. I have stood by him because of my commitment, loyalty and Christian faith. We were both active members of the church.

A couple of years ago, Mark started mucking around on the Internet. He could no longer work and I thought it was encouraging that he was stimulating his mind with information from the Net. I am completely computer illiterate and so was totally ignorant about what he was doing. Friends often asked me what he did online all day, but I just dismissed their concerns. No, he wasn't into pornography, I said. No, he hadn't met anyone else. Now, I think back to the many nights he said he couldn't sleep, and got out of bed so that he would not disturb me. I can now see that he was chatting. Without me even knowing it, he was becoming addicted to the Internet. He spent at least eight hours a day online while I went out and worked.

A couple of months ago, I commented to Mark that he looked unhappy. He casually brought up the idea that he should leave and let me get on with my life. I immediately thought he was depressed again, and sent him off to the doctor. The GP prescribed some anti-depressants and referred him to a clinical psychologist. At a joint session, Mark said that he wanted to set me free – to release me from the burden of taking care of him. It appeared to be very noble.

Six weeks later Mark told me that he loved me and that I had been a wonderful, devoted and faithful wife, but that he wasn't 'in love' with me. He said he didn't know if he ever was. He said that he wanted a trial separation to work himself out. Within one week, he had moved out. I was very distressed, but he was quite calm about the whole situation. I was worried how the kids would take it, and how he would manage on his own.

Five weeks after he had moved out, I found out that Mark

was organising a new passport. I confronted him about it. He admitted that he had met someone overseas. He had never met her [in person], but was planning to spend the rest of his life with her and her daughter. He swore that he had only met her [on the Internet] after he had left, but I quickly realised that this affair had been going on for some time. Looking back, it all made sense – it was like putting together the pieces of a jigsaw puzzle.

Mark told me that Susan appreciated him for who he was. She loved him for who he was, not who he could have been. He had met her in a chat room where he was counselling another woman who was upset about something. Susan was drawn to his sensitivity. I think she was drawn to a ticket to Australia. After I got over the initial shock, I was furious. After looking after him for seven years, he was going to walk out on me and the kids and walk into an instant family. I couldn't work out what would make a mother take her daughter away from the US, her family, friends and school, for a severely disabled man she had never met?

Now, I am no longer angry. I think he's a fool. I have already found out that she has been lying to him about various personal details. He is in fantasy land. Nothing he learns about her worries him. He feels that she is the right woman for him. How can she be? He has never met her. I feel I can slowly let go of him. I have no guilt. I stuck by him when he needed me, and he left me anyway. I would have stayed with him until his dying day. She flatters his deflated ego.

I can't believe that he has changed all his values and beliefs. He will not listen to anyone and has lost all his friends. He's listening to his Internet friends who tell him to follow his heart.

My main distress is for the children. They are having counselling and are very upset. They have begun to lose respect for him. They can't understand why he would choose a woman and her daughter who are strangers over them and me. I know he will fall flat on his face and that he may want to come back. The children will want me to take him back, but I can't. Too much has happened. I feel a sense of release. I am ready to get on with my life, and hopefully find another partner at some point. For now, I will just concentrate on getting the kids through this difficult time. ▶

Postscript – Two months later, I have found out that he is going overseas. He's going to argue in a US court that he'll be a fit father, financially and emotionally, for Susan's daughter. The father is trying to stop Susan taking their daughter to Australia. Mark is abandoning his own children to chase a new family he hasn't even met. ◄

We suggest that our society's ethical and moral guidelines have not yet caught up with technology. The rules of Internet relationships have yet to be prescribed. Our belief is that Internet relationships are no different than conventional affairs. Affairs are not just about physical sex, they are about betrayal, lies, deceit, rejection and lack of commitment. That conventional sex has not yet occurred and may never occur in Internet liaisons is irrelevant. It gets down to the crude basics – if you're online with someone else, you cannot be committed to your partner in real life. It has to be said, though, that some Internet affairs do go on to become real-life affairs.

▶ Daniel's story (43 years)

My wife has met someone on the Net. I suspected something was up because she became distant and always seemed to be picking on me. Finally I worked up the courage to check her emails (given she's always online) and sure enough, there were love letters from some guy in the UK.

She's younger than I am and we've been married for a long time. Our children are teenagers now and she says that she's sick of being everyone else's slave and regrets not having done anything with her life. She believes this man in England will offer her what has been missing in her own life. They haven't even met, though she tells me he knows her more intimately than I ever have. She's planning on visiting him at Christmas and who knows what after that. I'm devastated but also really shell-shocked. I can't believe that she will leave me for someone she hasn't even met in person. What can I do? ◄

If you are worried that your partner may be having an Internet affair, look through this list:

 Warning signs that your partner may be involved with someone on the Internet

- is online for long periods of time
- is secretive about their Internet use
- wants to be alone when they are using the computer
- shows less interest in you and your shared activities
- has less time for the children
- neglects regular household chores
- stays up very late or gets up very early to go online
- loses interest in your physical relationship
- seems preoccupied or 'unavailable' for you emotionally
- has unexplained credit card expenses or large telephone bills
- is secretive about the telephone or credit card bills
- leaves the computer on for long periods of time while doing other tasks around the house (waiting for instant messages)
- talks about travelling
- talks about having missed out on a lot of things in life
- discusses people they have met online

If you are reading our book as a user and are unsure as to whether you are crossing the boundary with someone online, answer the questions below.

Irrespective of which side of the Internet fence you are on, you need to get informed and take action. Internet problems will not go away unless you do something about them. If you are online with someone else, you need to make some difficult decisions. If

Is your Internet relationship getting out of hand?

- Do you long to tell your Internet partner rather than your actual partner about something exciting in your life?
- Does the communication you share online take up valuable time you could be spending with your partner, children, friends or on your own activities?
- Do you communicate mostly with one special person online?
- Are you aware of when they will be online?
- Do you try to think of ways you might be able to physically meet your Internet partner?
- Have you ever engaged in cyber sex with your Internet partner?
- Would you feel down if you were unable to correspond with your Internet partner for a period of time?

your partner's online with another person then you have to decide what course of action you will take. We'll look at what you can do about your situation in the next chapter.

N E W S F L A S H

A Japanese firm has designed a virtual girlfriend, who is attracting the attention of thousands of men. Men can pay a monthly fee to have a relationship with this fantasy woman, who replies to emails with messages generated by a computer program. The success of the relationship is measured by how many of her secrets the man can uncover and what percentage of her virtual heart he wins by asking the appropriate questions.

The Sydney Morning Herald 20/1/01

Other effects on your relationship

Think about your own life: which aspect of the Internet causes conflict in your relationship? Is it working at home in the evening to catch up on what you didn't have time for at the office, browsing on the Net, or spending time playing games? Each one of these in and of itself is certainly not a problem. They only become a problem when they remove you from other important activities in your relationship or cause tension. If your partner is upset about your behaviour then it is a problem for them. Because of your commitment to your partner, it is a good idea to listen to your partner's complaint. Or maybe your use of adult pornography, online gambling or shopping is getting out of hand and causing problems.

Working from home

We think that the Internet allows the boundaries between work and pleasure to become blurred, in much the same way as the mobile telephone has done over the past several years. Now it's: *I've just got to check my emails* or *I just have to look something up for work before bed.* What tends to happen is that a vicious cycle is set in motion. While one partner is online doing work, the other is feeling annoyed or unhappy because they're thinking that this is their time as a couple: *What about us?* From then on, it can go downhill as one thinks the other is unreasonable, and the other thinks they are being neglected. But as with all things, it's up to the individual to set their own limits, and this can be hard to do. Being flexible also helps relationships stay on track. In reality, though, if one of you spends a large amount of time online for work at home, and your partner is unhappy about it, you need to address the issue head-on. Don't let it fester. You certainly need to put in the hours to have quality couple time, so work out an arrangement that meets both your needs.

The upside, however, is that the Internet makes it possible to work from home during business hours if needed and this can be fabulous. Having workplace flexibility benefits companies and employees alike.

> ▶ **Trish's story [41 years]**
>
> Generally, Tom and I get on very well. We have been together for eighteen years. We have just got to the point where the kids do their own thing at night and we can relax. The trouble is we never spend any time together at night anymore. I am either watching television or reading a book, and Tom is on the computer. The same thing happens most nights. He says after dinner, 'I'll just quickly check my emails.' He then doesn't come out of the study for another two hours. I go in there every now and then to see what he's doing. But he's just reading or typing and tells me he won't be long. After a while, I just give up and go to bed. He wonders why our sex life has deteriorated, but if he is going to put the computer before me all the time, it's not my fault.
>
> Any time I have confronted him about it, he doesn't seem to think it is a problem. I remind him that before we had email, work would finish at 7 p.m. Now, there are no limits. It's as if he's on-call all the time. I don't know how we are going to solve this problem, because I'm the only one who thinks it's an issue. ◀

Couple differences

Tension can also arise within couples if one of you is absolutely enthralled by the Internet and the other isn't. Or maybe one of you has just had more time to learn about it. What develops between you, however, is a discrepancy in your understanding or exposure to the Net. The consequences of this might include conflict about the time you spend online and the money it costs. If these differences aren't managed effectively problems may arise.

We would suggest you try to bridge the gap between you. There are books to read and courses to take if you don't know much about the Internet. If you use the Internet a lot involve your partner, but at the same time check to see whether you need to put some limits in place. 'Know when to get offline' and 'Get informed, take action' are two of our conclusions that are relevant to you both.

Online games and surfing

In much the same way as working from home can cause problems in relationships, so can excessive game-playing and information-browsing on the Net. For people who want stimulation the Internet provides the perfect medium. As we've said before, the Internet is always open and easily accessible. Again it comes back to knowing when to get offline – danger lies ahead for those who find it hard to put on their own brakes.

Pornography

The use of pornography or erotica is, by and large, a male thing. Though having said that, many women enjoy the use of it in their relationship. Before the Internet there were the typical 'girlie' magazines, pin-up calendars, blue movies and strip clubs. Now we have all of these plus the Internet. Adult pornography is big business; adult pornography on the Internet is big business – so much so that in one recent interview on US television, the star of an adult site reported 13 million hits to her site per day. By logging on and paying a fee, users can view the material on offer.

While the use of pornography is not new, what's different is the availability and accessibility to it via the Internet. The risk of some of you becoming hooked on it is greater than in the pre-Internet days because you don't have to work as hard to reap the rewards. Gone are the days of going to your local newsagency to buy your favourite magazine, sheepishly renting an X-rated video at the store, or anonymously making a catalogue purchase of the latest material. Now with the push of a few buttons, you can view whatever you like, whenever you like, all in the privacy of your home.

For some couples, the use of pornography isn't an issue. For others it is a great source of tension. How you think about the use of erotic material in your own relationship will depend on a whole range of issues, including how you think about yourself, your partner, the message you believe is behind such images, and whether you find the material offensive.

▶ Doug's story [39 years]

People ask me why my marriage broke down. I find it hard to answer them. To me, there were lots of reasons – we stopped having any fun, we stopped having sex, we stopped talking. If you were to ask Rachel, though, she would say that we broke up because I was looking at pornography on the Internet.

We had been married for ten years, together for fourteen. Yes, it was wonderful at first. I thought I'd found my soul mate. We had so much in common and laughed at so much. We weren't able to start a family, but we were okay with that. Neither of us wanted to go down the IVF path. We seemed happy with our life together and made many plans for our future. After we had been married for about eight years, Rachel started to talk about feeling as if she was missing something in her life. I thought she was talking about children, but she reassured me that she wasn't. She said that she just didn't feel as if she was achieving anything. I didn't understand what she meant, because she was very successful in her career. She started to withdraw from that point. She spent more time with girlfriends and wasn't interested in anything I suggested we do.

I became lonely. I had always done a bit of work at home at night, but on the many nights I spent at home alone, I really started to miss her. One night, I was on the Net and I just looked up a few porn sites. They didn't really impress me, but they didn't repulse me either. The next time I was at home alone, I revisited these sites. I started to look forward to the nights when Rachel was out, so that I could look at these sites. It didn't take long before I would start getting restless if I couldn't get on the Net in privacy. I no longer did much work at night, I spent hours and hours looking at porn. I knew it wasn't healthy for my marriage, because I no longer cared if Rachel and I had sex or not. There was nothing I could do to stop my behaviour though, I was hooked.

Everything came crashing down when Rachel came home one night when she was meant to be out. She caught me masturbating in front of the screen and was mortified. She hurled all sorts of abuse at me and practically ended the marriage on the spot. ◖▸◗

> At the time, I felt very guilty and took on all the responsibility of the break-up. But now, I look back at the times leading up to that night and I know there was a lot more to it. But I guess if I hadn't been hooked on the pornography, I would have made more of an effort to save our marriage. ◄

It's not uncommon then to see the issue snowball, especially if the one using the pornography is secretive about it. For many women, they start to take personally their partner's actions: *What's wrong with me? If I was enough he'd have no need to look at pictures of other women.* But men don't see it that way – it's something different for them, something totally separate from their partner.

If it is a problem for her, the mere act of logging on to the computer can set off a chain reaction of suspicion, insecurity and conflict. The bottom line is that the relationship suffers, and without an effective way to manage the situation the relationship is placed in jeopardy. Even though his behaviour doesn't constitute an affair, it is still having a negative impact on the relationship, and something needs to change.

▶ Patty's story [38 years]

I would say that we have a pretty good marriage. We are a little team and help and support each other. We have three children and so are pretty busy. We do spend quite a lot of time together as a family and as a couple. Our sex life isn't what it used to be, but I have no real complaints.

My husband doesn't know that I know he visits all these pornographic sites. I go to bed earlier than he does because I am so tired, and he works on the computer at night. I only found out by accident because I was trying to find something on the Net. I knew that he had looked up the same thing recently and so I clicked on the History icon. Up came the addresses of these sites and so I had a look. I was shocked at first, not because I am disgusted by pornography but because I didn't know about it. We talk very openly about things and so I would have thought that he would talk to me about his desire to use pornography.

I haven't said anything to him, but I do worry about it. I can't help wondering if he is unsatisfied with our sex life, and whether the next step is for him to have an affair or go to a prostitute. I can't bring myself to confront him about it yet, but I know I will have to because it is eating away at me. I would have to say that I have been more withdrawn from him since I found out. ◀

If you are in a relationship with someone whose use of pornography concerns you, the strategies we outline in the next chapter may give you some ideas about how to approach the subject. If you believe your own use of pornography is an issue in your relationship then you will most likely benefit from reading Chapter 8 and our self-help program for excessive Internet use in Chapter 9.

Compulsive online gambling and shopping

Some of you reading this book will believe you have a problem with gambling or shopping online, or are concerned about someone close to you. Some of the danger signs include:

- you feel a strong urge to go online to gamble or shop
- you feel helpless to stop your behaviour
- you have tried to cut back without success
- you have lied to those close to you about your activities
- you are in debt
- you have risked your relationship or job because of your behaviour
- you feel guilty about your online behaviour

Obviously the impact on your life and those closest to you can be great. You have a lot to lose both financially and personally. If you think you have a problem then admitting it is the first step. Seeking appropriate help is the second. Read through our self-help program in Chapter 9. We would then encourage you to contact a health professional who specialises in the treatment of compulsive gambling or compulsive shopping. It's probably too hard to do it on your own, especially if it has been going on for a long time. If you are concerned about your partner, we would recommend you encourage them to seek help. If they won't go, go yourself.

In brief...

- More and more relationships are being threatened by Internet romances.
- Internet affairs *are* affairs.
- The boundaries between work and home life can be blurred by the ease of the Internet.
- Relationships can suffer because of other Internet activities including game-playing, surfing the Net and online pornography, gambling and shopping.

The Lighter Side...

Dear Tech Support,

Last year I upgraded from Boyfriend 5.0 to Husband 1.0 and noticed that the new program began making unexpected changes to the accounting modules, limiting access to flower and jewellery applications that had operated flawlessly under Boyfriend 5.0. In addition, Husband 1.0 uninstalled many other valuable programs, such as Romance 9.9 but installed undesirable programs such as NFL 5.0 and NBA 3.0. Conversation 8.0 no longer runs and HouseCleaning 2.6 simply crashes the system. I've tried running Nagging 5.3 to fix these problems, but to no avail.

Desperate

Dear Desperate,

Keep in mind, Boyfriend 5.0 is an entertainment package, while Husband 1.0 is an operating system. Try to enter the command: C:/ I THOUGHT YOU LOVED ME and install Tears 6.2. Husband 1.0 should then automatically run the applications: Guilty 3.0 and Flowers 7.0. But remember, overuse can cause Husband 1.0 to default to Grumpy Silence 2.5, Happy Hour 7.0 or Beer 6.1. Beer 6.1 is a very bad program that will create 'Snoring Loudly' wave files. DO NOT install MotherInLaw 1.0 or reinstall another Boyfriend program. These are not supported applications and will crash Husband 1.0.

In summary, Husband 1.0 is a great program, but it does have limited memory and cannot learn new applications quickly. Consider buying additional software to improve performance. I personally recommend HotFood 3.0 and Lingerie 5.3.

Tech Support

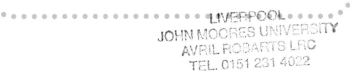

5

Help for committed relationships

We've looked at how Internet relationships differ from conventional ones and how they mimic the intense first phase of a new relationship. In the previous chapter we explained why we believe Internet affairs are affairs and how they threaten commitment in a relationship. Now we want to turn your attention to what you need to do to get your marriage back on track if either one of you is caught in the web of an Internet relationship. We make a number of suggestions for those of you who are involved with someone on the Net and if your partner is online with someone else.

Caught between the two

If you have met someone on the Net and believe your feelings for them are affecting your committed relationship, you have an important decision to make – and the earlier the better. The key to getting your life back on track with your real-life partner is commitment. Our definition sees commitment as a mindset or a way of thinking that gets played out in everyday life. It's about making sure your behaviour reflects the fact that you have chosen to be with your partner for the rest of your life. If you are spending time online with a specific person or certain types of people then you are not committed. Some of you may criticise us for this strong stance, but ask yourself: *Do you hide anything that you do online from your partner?* Even if they never ask you and you never volunteer information about what you do, ask yourself: *Would they mind if they knew?* If the answers to these questions are 'yes', admitting you have a problem is the first step on the path to re-establishing your commitment to your partner.

What do you do?

After you admit to yourself that your involvement with your Internet partner is affecting your committed relationship, then the hard work begins. In Chapter 4 we asked you to complete 'Is your Internet relationship getting out of hand?' If you haven't answered the questions then have a go now. If you answered 'yes' to any of these questions then read on as you now need to focus your attention on issues in your own relationship. You may not want to hear this, but breaking off your Internet relationship, irrespective of what form it takes, is your only choice if you are to remain on your relationship path.

We have summarised our suggestions below and recommend that you write down your answers to the exercises as you go.

 Steps to bring your Internet affair to an end

1. Write down your answers to 'Is your Internet relationship getting out of hand?' (see Chapter 4).
2. Consider the likely consequences for yourself, your partner and your children if you were to continue in your Internet relationship. ▶

3. Stop your Internet contact immediately.

4. Start working on identifying any problems in your relationship that need to be addressed.

5. Reaffirm your commitment to your partner.

6. Make sure your behaviour reflects this commitment – and that means giving up the Internet liaison.

Let's now take a closer look at what's involved in each step.

1. Write down the answers to 'Is your Internet relationship getting out of hand?'

We always ask our clients to write down their thoughts about certain things because a lot more cognitive processing is involved when you put pen to paper. It's important to be honest with yourself otherwise you'll end up making decisions based on inaccurate information.

2. Consider the likely consequences for yourself, your partner and your children if you were to continue in your Internet relationship

Thinking about the consequences of your behaviour helps you make an informed decision. To help you do this, write down your answers to the following:

- What is likely to happen for me if I continue communicating with X?
- How will this affect my partner?
- What is likely to happen to our relationship?
- How will this affect my children?

3. Stop your Internet contact immediately

We can hear many of you saying: *That's easier said than done.* Like any behaviour that is pleasurable, it's going to be hard to give it up. So we suggest you decide to cease all contact for the next week while you work through this chapter. If you really want to get your relationship back on track, your behaviour needs to match your thinking.

4. Start working on identifying any problems in your relationship that need to be addressed

Often when people look elsewhere for intimacy they avoid looking inwards at their own behaviour within their relationship. Remember that the perfect relationship doesn't exist; there is no saint or angel. If you were being totally honest with yourself and your partner, list the issues about which you have been unhappy.

We strongly believe that if an issue is worrying you it is your responsibility to raise it with your partner. Maybe you have been unhappy with your sexual relationship, the amount of time you spend together or how you communicate. Regardless of the issues that have resulted in you getting close to someone else, you need to go back to your partner and have a serious discussion with them. We refer to this as 'owning your problem'. If you've been complaining about your partner to someone on the Net, or anyone else for that matter, that is your cue to stop talking to others, and talk to your partner. Your partner will not be able to read your mind, so you must tell them your concerns. If you find talking to your partner quite awkward, you might benefit from our OCEAN model of communication (outlined later in this chapter). You do need to think ahead of time about the issues you want to discuss, and what changes you'd like to see happen.

If you're having trouble working out exactly what your issues are then ask yourself: *What needs are being met by my Internet partner that aren't being met by my partner?* Some people say their e-partner is always there for them, or listens to them or seems interested in what they do each day. To improve your relationship you need to be clear about the issues – hopefully, by now you are. If not, think back to some recent times when you felt angry or upset with your partner. What was it about? The following questions may give you some clues.

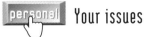 **Your issues**

- What are the typical issues that cause conflict or tension in your relationship?
- What aspects of your relationship make you sad or angry?
- What do you think is missing in your relationship?
- What would you change about it if you could?
- What do you think is missing in your own life?
- What would you do differently if you could have your time over again?

5. Reaffirm your commitment to your partner

Giving up your Internet partner won't be easy. It is crucial to be clear in your own mind why you are choosing to end the relationship and acknowledge that it is your choice. If you are only giving it up because you think you should, we wouldn't be very confident in your ability to follow through. Your commitment to your partner is the key – you made a decision to spend your life with your partner. Presumably you believed you were good together back then. Think back to what first attracted you to your partner? Even though it may be hard to remember, you and your partner were once in the bubble of new love too. How did you feel? What did you do?

 You and your partner

- What first attracted you to your partner?
- How did it feel to be in the bubble of new love?
- What did you do together in those early days?

You need to tell your partner that you are reconfirming your commitment. That might mean being totally up front if they know about your Internet liaison. If they don't know, you might need to first talk about how you think you've become unstuck lately and want to get your relationship back on track.

6. Make sure your behaviour reflects this commitment – and that means giving up the Internet liaison

Hopefully by now you understand why you need to give up your Internet relationship if you want to continue in your committed relationship. If you don't, ask yourself how you would feel if your partner was having an Internet affair? If you still think you can have your cake and eat it too, you need to consider deciding to end your marriage, because you're not committed. We call people who want to have both relationships 'cake eaters'. We strongly advise anyone to end a relationship with a cake eater because a relationship is doomed without commitment.

> ▶ **Tim's story [27 years]**
>
> A friend shared his experience after seeing the effect the Internet had had on his family. His parents had been married for 28 years and had four children. After his parents bought a computer and connected to the Internet his mum became interested in chat rooms after she saw her children talking to people all around the world.
>
> Soon she became a regular user and was staying up often until 3 a.m. talking to people in chat rooms. These were often men from many different countries. She was excited by this experience and shared stories of the people with whom she chatted. The more her husband heard, the more uncomfortable and jealous he became. The tension grew between them and arguments were becoming frequent.
>
> The children were concerned about their parents' relationship, fearing that they'd split up. They decided to talk to their

parents about their concerns. Only then did the mother realise she must stop chatting online to resolve the ongoing conflict with her husband. Tim was relieved to see his parents' relationship start to mend. ◀

How to end your Internet affair

Let's now look at three techniques that may help you stick to your decision to end your Internet relationship.

1. Your partner's shoes

We often see the partners of those involved in an Internet relationship before we see the people themselves, if at all. The partners tend to be distressed, confused and at a loss as to what action they need to take. If you're having an Internet relationship, it is important to have some understanding of how your partner might be feeling. To do this, we ask our clients to put themselves in their partner's shoes, to feel empathy, and so understand a little of what their partner might be feeling. Try the following exercise.

 ## Put yourself in your partner's shoes

Imagine your partner is always on the Net. Maybe you know they're intimately communicating with someone else, maybe you don't. Your hunch is that they are. But what you do know is lately they've become distant, they don't seem very interested in you anymore. They're tired and irritable and snap at you. They really don't want to get too close to you at all. You feel confused; a mixture of sadness, anger and helplessness. You ask them what's going on, but they fob you off. You ask again and again, but still you are none the wiser.

○ How do you think you might feel?

- What if they then started talking about leaving you and had not given you a chance to fight for your relationship?
- How do you think you might feel then?

Obviously you won't and can't ever imagine what someone else is thinking or feeling, but putting yourself in your partner's shoes is perhaps as close as you can get to having a sense of what they're experiencing. Asking them how they are thinking and feeling without defending yourself will also help you see it from their point of view.

2. Clear thinking

We talk in Chapter 9 about the importance of changing unhelpful thinking patterns when you're trying to manage excessive Internet use. If you want to end an Internet relationship, the same strategies can help you manage the difficult process of breaking the connection (literally). It's important to ensure that your thinking is constructive and supports the decision you have made to end your Internet liaison.

If you start doubting your ability to stick with your decision to cease all contact with your e-partner, it might help you to say to yourself:

I want to remain in my relationship with my partner because of a, b and c. I can't do this if I continue to be involved on the Net with X. I wouldn't like it if our roles were reversed – I can't have my cake and eat it too. It's going to be difficult but I'm choosing to stay.

Or:

I will miss my contact with X, but if I choose to keep up our communication then I am not putting in 100 percent to my relationship. I'll take it one day at a time and start focusing on rebuilding my relationship with my partner.

If you find you are having unhelpful thoughts about your situation, we suggest you keep a record of those thoughts and challenge them in the way we outline in Chapter 9, using the A-B-C-D-E diary format.

3. Close the door firmly

Be clear to your Internet partner; be direct about the reasons why you are choosing to end the relationship, and close the door firmly. By that we mean cease all contact. You and your real-life partner need to know the contact has stopped so there is no room for doubt and suspicion. Prepare what you want to say or write to your e-partner. The following might give you a few ideas.

> *I've been thinking about our relationship a lot and realise that over the past months I've neglected my partner. Our contact is jeopardising my commitment to my relationship and I don't want to lose him/her, so I've made the decision to end all our contact. I'm sorry for any pain I've caused but my relationship is my number one priority. Please don't contact me in any way.*

You may need to be prepared for a negative reaction from your Internet partner. Work out an action plan ahead of time if you suspect trouble. Obviously all situations will vary, depending on where you each live, how much personal information you've disclosed and whether you've met in person. You may, for example, need to change your email address. If your ex-Internet partner starts to harass you, you'll need to do something about it. We understand that if something happens on the Net that would constitute a crime in real life, it's still a crime.

If you do leave your relationship

If throughout the process of ending your Internet relationship you realise you do not want to remain in your marriage, you need to make that decision and move on. We recommend you make an informed decision based on facts not feelings. Have you tried every option to get your relationship back on track, including counselling? You need to think about the consequences of leaving.

Where will you go? What about your children? What about your financial situation? Once you walk out the door it is very hard to walk back in and pick up where you left off. It is certainly not a decision to be made lightly.

We strongly recommend that you don't pursue a real-life relationship with your Internet partner immediately, otherwise you are setting yourself up to fail. We believe people need time on their own once their relationship has ended regardless of whether they were the one who left or not. You need time to look at where the relationship went wrong so you are less likely to make the same mistakes again.

Before you enter into any new relationship, we recommend the ground rules listed below. If you use the Internet a lot to meet people then the last ground rule is very important: ***Don't restrict yourself to meeting people online.*** Even though it may be hard because the Net is easy for you and you are familiar with it, we would encourage you to get out and meet people in lots of places. Go to all the conventional haunts such as work functions, courses, sporting clubs and friends' parties. Don't turn down social invitations. It's important that the Net is only one part of your life, not your whole life.

 Ground rules for starting a new relationship

- Take a long break.
- Make friends not lovers.
- Date different people.
- Take your time.
- Don't rush into sex.
- Tell yourself that it is okay to be single for a while.
- Seek counselling if necessary.
- Don't restrict yourself to meeting people online.

If you are considering a real-life relationship with your e-partner, we suggest you keep in mind the guidelines for developing an Internet relationship in Chapter 3. You especially need time together in everyday life to discover each other's warts, and to work out whether your online feelings materialise into physical chemistry. It is important to keep your thinking realistic about your e-partner, especially if you believe they are a saint or angel. Remember our second conclusion – take your time approaching anyone or anything online. To do this you need to keep your thinking in check. It might help to tell yourself something like:

> *I know it feels like we know each other very well, but until we have spent a reasonable amount of time together we don't really know how we'll get on. We need to take it slowly and do things together as though we had just met yesterday, because I suppose in a way we have.*

If you haven't met your Internet partner in real life yet, you haven't had an opportunity to uncover any lies. Unfortunately, they still can be anyone they like at this stage. Don't fall into the trap of thinking you've now found greener grass – you may have found grass that is indeed much browner.

If your partner is involved with someone on the Net

If you've read this book from the beginning, you probably by now have a better feel for Internet relationships. If your partner is intimately involved with people on the Net, or one person in particular, you no doubt feel helpless, confused and angry. How you manage this situation will have a lot to do with how your partner is treating you and what you've been told about their Internet liaisons. We encourage people in your position to find ways to increase your sense of control over the situation. How, you might ask? We'll show you how throughout the rest of this chapter.

▶ Pete's story (44 years)

Deborah and I explored chat rooms together, just for fun. We were given the address of a room that we were told would be a bit of a laugh. That's all I thought it was – harmless fun. One day, I started chatting to a woman in Queensland who was married with three kids. It didn't take long before she was telling me that she loved me and wanted to send me the money for me to fly up and be with her. I was shocked. That was before I knew what Deborah had been doing.

I started having my suspicions about Deborah having met someone on the Net about one month after she had met Stuart. She kept talking about this guy all the time. She talked about lots of people she had met on the Internet, but his name came up more often. She talked to a number of people she had met online on the phone. One time, when I walked in on her talking to Stuart, she said 'Stuart wants to talk to you' and he started calling me his mate and being very friendly. I wasn't fooled. I knew there was something going on. So I spent $3500 on monitors to find out what was happening. I had a unit set up on my Internet line so I could replay all the chatting that was going on. I also had the phone bugged and listened to all the calls. This was how I found out that Deborah was apparently in love with Stuart. They were even engaged! She planned to leave me and take our son to be with Stuart in America. He was planning to leave his wife – or so he said.

When I confronted Deborah, she admitted that she loved Stuart and didn't love me. She said she had been to a solicitor to see about a divorce, and passport documents for our son. At that point, I was not shocked, but very hurt. I thought hard about letting her go but there was no way I was going to let her take our son.

[But] because I loved her, I couldn't let her go without trying to show her what a mistake she was making. I first got a block put on our son's passport so she couldn't take him anywhere. Then I set about investigating the new love of her life. I enlisted the help of the NYPD, ASIO and Interpol. They were all very helpful, but could not lay any charges against him, as having an Internet affair is not a crime. I found out with the help of these agencies that Stuart is pending trial on criminal charges. This was the man my wife was going to leave me for! I believe that if I hadn't uncovered the truth, she would have gone.

Two weeks after I confronted Deborah, we went to counselling. The counsellor advised us that Deborah had to discover for herself that the Internet was not good for her. I left my job so that I could watch what she was up to. As a result of being unemployed, we gave up on the dream home we had been building. I had to give our marriage top priority.

I am trying to trust Deborah again, but it is very difficult. She has continued to lie to me and even kept talking to him at first. I get very depressed at times. I want things to get better between us, but it will never be as good as it used to be. I thought we had a good marriage. If Deborah had problems, she should have come to me about them – not turn to a complete stranger. I don't think Deborah's actions were any better than Stuart's.

I tried to talk to the operators of the chat room about their duty of care to their customers. From then on, they banned Deborah and me from the chat room. I only hope something good can come about as a result of all this. That is why I have set up my own investigation company, and why I am writing to government ministers seeking their assistance. I am planning to set up a victims' support group some time down the track, because there must be many people in the same boat as us.

My heart has had a chunk taken out of it as I have never cheated on her. I feel that anything she may say to me has no meaning. Given what I know about her past and her cheating, I firmly believe that she is her own worst enemy. ◄

▶ Deborah's story [36 years]

Everything blew up with Pete in mid-September. At the time, I told Pete that I didn't love him and that I loved Stuart and wanted to be with him. It was only after Pete started to find out that Stuart had lied about everything and that he was very inconsistent in his stories, that I began to realise who I had fallen in love with. ▶

He had lied about his job and was talking to many women from all over the world.

Pete and I went to counselling, but I didn't find it to be very helpful. The counsellor was telling me that it was all right for me to keep using the chat rooms and that I should go to my local library if Pete had the home line tapped. Pete was telling me that I was hooked on the Internet and that I should have learnt that I needed to stay away from it. I was confused. I wanted my marriage to work, but it was very hard to give up my addiction. These people had become part of my life and I felt sad to give them up – especially Stuart.

Looking back, I don't know what I was thinking. It was all so fast, so intense. I am not an emotionally disturbed person. Just because I don't show my feelings to Pete doesn't mean that I don't love him and that I am not sorry for what I have done.

I want to work on the marriage. I no longer talk in the chat rooms. I have no contact with my Internet friends or Stuart. I am so embarrassed about what has happened and how silly I have been. I have learnt a lesson. I only hope Pete can get past this and stop throwing it back at me all the time. I can't undo the past, and reminding me about it all the time doesn't help us to move on. ◀

It's easy to see from Pete and Deborah's stories the damage that can be done to relationships by Internet affairs. They are working actively on getting their marriage back on track even though they have used some extreme measures. Knowing where to start if your partner is having an e-relationship is usually a tough question. Let's look at what you can do.

What you can do about their relationship

There are five important areas for you to concentrate on when tackling the problem at hand. These are: seek support, don't neglect the danger signs, own the problem, build a new relationship and seek professional help. We also outline our OCEAN model of communication in the section on owning your problem, as this is a useful framework to use when expressing yourself.

1. Seek support

The first step you must take is for you. As soon as you seriously think that your partner is involved with someone on the Net, find yourself a support network. Whether you turn to a friend, a health professional or a support group, it is important to have someone you can confide in as you most likely will be riding an emotional roller coaster for some time. Seeking legal advice might also be warranted where children are involved so as to prevent your children being taken out of the country, for example, without your permission.

2. Don't neglect the warning signs

We listed in Chapter 4 a number of warning signs that may alert you to the fact that your partner is having an Internet relationship. Don't bury your head in the sand. Familiarise yourself with these signs, as they aren't all going to be obvious on day one.

Some people who start having Internet affairs go on to have real-life affairs with their Internet partner. At this point, you might be even more confused as your partner's behaviour will change, and so will the warning signs. For example, their Internet use will most likely drastically reduce, and their time away from home will increase.

3. Own the problem

By owning the problem we mean acknowledging that your partner's behaviour on the Internet is a problem *for you*. Your partner probably thinks they are doing nothing wrong so it's up to you to bring it to their attention. If their behaviour is upsetting you, make a decision to let them know how you feel. You can't expect them to mind read what is bugging you.

Owning the problem and then bringing up your issues is a huge step in taking control of the situation. Before you discuss your partner's Internet use with them, you need to be clear about what you want to ask them to do differently. It's important not to rush in and blurt out your anger and hurt. That's why being able to diffuse your feelings with a friend or therapist is helpful. Decide what behaviours you will and won't tolerate. If you don't really know what your partner is up to on the Net, work on what you do know; stick to the facts. They can't refute, for example, that they're online for six hours each night and are neglecting their family duties or your relationship. If you accuse them of every sordid scenario you've read about then it is all too easy for them to lose sight of what the real issues are, by dismissing all of your allegations at once.

When you are ready to confront your partner about their behaviour, tell them you'd like to talk about their Internet use, and set a mutually agreeable time; a time and place when you won't be disturbed. Keep yourselves out of earshot of your children; it doesn't help them to hear what you will be discussing. Then follow the steps in our OCEAN model of communication, which we first described in *Side by Side*. We developed the OCEAN acronym as an easy way of remembering the steps needed to address any problem. The key is to be able to express to your partner how you feel about their Internet use, and how you'd like them to change. Once you start tackling the problem in this way it's hard to say where it will end up. But a lack of commitment is at the heart of what you're experiencing. The bottom line is: if your partner is communicating intimately with someone on the Net, they are not committed to you. Whether they will change their behaviour is their decision.

N E W S F L A S H

Some people are setting up web cams in their homes so that they can monitor what is going on there while at work. A recent case involved a young man who came home to find that his flat had been burgled. He was able to post images of the two intruders on the Net, and invited people to identify them.

The Sydney Morning Herald 2/01

The OCEAN model of communication

O = Own the problem

C = Change unhelpful thinking

E = Express the problem

A = Ask for help assertively

N = Negotiate

O = Own the problem

Owning the problem is the most important step as nobody else will be able to fix it for you. If you have not owned the problem, there is not much hope of a satisfying resolution.

C = Change unhelpful thinking

Many of your distressing feelings can be put down to the unhelpful way you think at times. It's really important to stick with the facts about your partner's Internet use. Keep away from thoughts such as: *What if she's in love and is going to leave me?* Until you know this for sure, it doesn't help you in your attempt to salvage your relationship.

E = Express the problem

Now you are in a position to express your problem. Remember, the aim is to let your partner know how unhappy you are about their Internet behaviour. Stay calm and don't attack them. Be prepared for the fact that your partner may not yet be ready to admit to you, or to themselves for that matter, that their Internet behaviour is a problem. Plan what you want to say before you meet. If your partner refuses to ever listen to you, you've got a very serious problem to face. At the end of this chapter we suggest what to do when you hit a brick wall like this.

A = Ask for help assertively

Requesting help is very difficult but essential. When doing so it is important to be assertive. Assertiveness can be defined as telling someone the truth in an appropriate manner. By 'an appropriate manner', we mean you do not see yourself as superior to others, perhaps leading to aggressive behaviour. Neither does it mean that you see yourself as inferior to others, which can lead to passive behaviour. It just means that you see yourself as equal to others.

A general rule of thumb is to use 'I' statements in your request. Starting a discussion with 'You' ... inevitably causes the other person to get defensive and start a fight or refuse to talk. Remember, your partner is already likely to be on the defensive. But starting a discussion with 'I' ... increases the likelihood that the other person will listen to whatever problem you have. Making a request moves your situation one step closer to working out a resolution, one way or another. Here is an example of owning the problem, expressing it and asking for help:

'I really don't like you chatting with that English guy. I'm feeling very insecure about us and would like you to stop your relationship with him completely.'

N = Negotiate

Negotiation is needed in all relationships at some stage. If you and your partner can't agree on the appropriateness of their Internet behaviour, you have to sit down and work out a solution that is agreeable to you both. In the OCEAN model, negotiation is the final step if your request for change is met with opposition.

4. Build a new relationship

If your partner decides to end their Internet contact, both of you have to work on getting your own relationship back on track. Your relationship will now be different from before – it has to be. Now is the time to put safeguards in place to prevent your relationship from heading down the slippery slope again. It's up to both of you to work on the issues that led one of you to get close to someone else. Some couples benefit from seeking professional help, others do it on their own. Regardless of whether you seek help or not, the following guidelines will help.

Guidelines for rebuilding after an Internet affair

To rebuild your relationship after an Internet affair, each of you needs to take the following steps.

The one who has had the Internet affair:

- Admit you were wrong to yourself and your partner.
- Cease all contact with the other person.
- Destroy all love letters, photos and other personal keepsakes.
- Change your contact details.
- Listen to your partner.
- Answer questions openly and honestly; keeping other facts hidden prevents you from beginning again with a clean slate.
- Work out where you went wrong: what issues in your relationship were you unhappy about? What did you neglect?
- Decide what limits you need to set in place to keep your own behaviour in check in the future.
- Recommit to your partner.
- Pay attention to your partner's needs.

The one who was on the receiving end:

- Expect to feel numb for some time, as you are going through a grieving process.
- Make an informed choice about whether or not you want to remain in your relationship.
- If you do want to stay, challenge unhelpful thinking that keeps you 'stuck' and rehashing the affair.
- Set a limit for when you will stop asking questions.

- Resist the urge to check your partner's computer for evidence that they might have resumed Internet contact.
- Build your own interests.
- Decide on what behaviour you will and won't tolerate.
- Work out where you think your relationship went wrong and what changes you would like to make.

Counselling may help prevent you both from repeating mistakes.

After any affair it will always take time to rebuild trust. Try to be patient, but decide to work hard at trusting your partner again.

online Ways of rebuilding trust

- Allow time to grieve.
- Make special time to spend together.
- Use clear thinking.
- Look for common goals.
- Learn to change your behaviour for the good of your relationship.

Having special time together is very relevant when the Internet has caused problems in your relationship. Typically, in the lead up to any revelation about an Internet affair, the amount of time you have spent together has been gradually whittled away because of the time one of you has spent online. Therefore, it is especially important to spend more time together. There should be many more hours free now if your partner has ceased all contact with their Internet partner. So be creative, do something you haven't done for years.

5. Seek professional help

If you get to the point where the two of you can't agree about your partner's Internet behaviour, we strongly suggest you seek professional help as a couple with a psychologist who is experienced in relationship issues and preferably has some understanding of the Internet. If your partner won't go with you, go alone. You will have some tough decisions ahead of you. If you have children and you are worried about your partner leaving the State or country, seek legal advice.

Hitting a brick wall

If you find you're at the point where your partner won't give up their Internet relationships or activities and you can't live with them, you've hit a brick wall. You need to decide how much longer you'll tolerate what they are doing. You might reach the point where you decide to leave, even if you have been committed all along. When this happens, it is very sad because it is beyond your control. Commitment is a two-way path and if there's only one of you on it then there is no relationship. If you believe you have exhausted all possibilities to get your partner to change their behaviour, you can walk away knowing that you tried everything to save your relationship.

In brief...

- If you want to remain in your relationship, cease all contact with your Internet partner.
- Speak up if your partner's online behaviour concerns you.
- You *can* rebuild your relationship after an Internet affair.

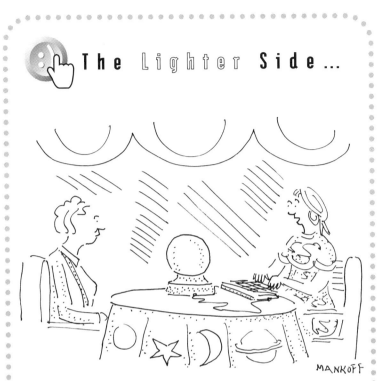

The Lighter Side...

"I've contacted your husband. He's at http://hottalk.com and wants to know what I look like naked."

‹6›

Teenagers on the Net

Many parents have approached us with their concerns about their children on the Internet. These concerns range from simple questions about how much time their children should be spending online, to grave worry about a relationship their teenager is having with somebody they met on the Internet. In this chapter, we will outline some of the issues teenagers face while on the Net. In the following chapter, we set out advice to concerned parents.

It is important to realise that there are lots of positives for teenagers on the Net. For example, teenagers who are geographically isolated can feel a greater sense of belonging due to the Internet. The Internet also allows the development of friendships without the influence of cultural, class and gender differences.

Teenagers (like everybody else) are talking on the Internet to people they already know, and don't know. Separate issues arise depending on which group of people they are talking to. There are some overlapping concerns, but we will try to deal with them separately, beginning with teenagers chatting to existing friends online.

Online with people they know

Ask any parent of older children and they'll tell you the teenage years are trying times. There have always been and will continue to be problems for parents of teenagers. The Internet provides another medium for the same old problems. It has also delivered parents of teenagers a whole new set of issues to deal with.

In the good ol' days

Once upon a time, teenagers would spend the entire night on the phone. They treated the home as a boarding house; home was somewhere to rest their weary bones after a busy night of socialising. Parents were worried then, frustrated then. Now, some can only wish things were this simple. Although teenagers got into trouble and were not concentrating on schoolwork and uni work, at least they were doing what normal teenagers do – making friends. These years from thirteen to nineteen are important in developing self-esteem through the learning of social skills. Teenagers need to rebel against their parents. They need to test the limits alone and with their friends. They learn a lot about themselves and get closer to their friends while testing the limits.

These same years see the development of skills in flirting and the discovery of sexuality. The awkward first kisses, sexual experiences and first love are all rites of passage for these young people. We are about to find out the consequences of losing the opportunity for such experiences, because now it is all changing.

And now ...

Now, many young people are spending more and more time online. They are chatting to their school friends and uni friends on the Net. It's all too easy to just log on and chat. It's instantaneous, ever accessible and so easy. Not much effort is needed and therefore not many skills are learnt. How can someone possibly learn the finer art of flirtation without face-to-face contact? The

ch@t

Dialogue – Teenagers		Comments
Hansard warning: Do not disclose your passwords or personal details while on chat. Protect yourself from Internet abuse.		*General warning is a great idea*
Rules: No offensive language, no repeating, no sexual attitudes, no cyber sex, no polling, no advertising, listen to channel hosts.		*Let's see if they follow the rules*
Dolly	> im bored. mikey u here talk 2 me plz	*Mikey, you here? Talk to me please*
XTC	> hi dolly	
Teenqueen	> any 1 want to chat	
Channel host	> **XTC, please change your nickname – not suitable for teens**	*Shows the host is watching*
XTC	> are u kidding me	
Channel host	> **nope. it's a drug reference**	
XTC	> it's also a feeling	*No respect for host*
Channel host	> **bad luck it's also a drug reference and not appropriate**	
Dolly	> how r we all	
Dreamboy	> im a good	
Dreamboy	> sorta	
Dolly	> lol	*lol = laugh out loud*
Dreamboy	> I will be in 2 secs	*Reference to masturbation*
Dolly	> thats good	
Dreamboy	> 1	
Dreamboy	> 2	
Dolly	> whats in 2 secs	*Shows Dolly doesn't realise what he's doing*
Dreamboy	> 3	
Channel host	> **not in here you're not**	*The channel host realises*
Dreamboy	> any second now	
Dreamboy	> yipppppppy	

Dolly	> lol	*Laugh out loud*
Dreamboy	> f**k your hot	*Not the best person for your daughter to be talking to*
Channel host	**> WARNING – no swearing or implied in teens**	*Attempt to enforce rules*
Dreamboy	> sorry	*Respect for channel host*
Maybebaby	> stats XTC	*Stats = statistics of person required*
XTC	> 15 m Syd	*Fifteen-year-old male from Sydney*
RUREADY	> stop asking me to go priv then talk to someone	*priv = private*
Dolly	> I didn't ask u 2 go priv	
RUREADY	> not you	
Dolly	> get over it	
Channel host	**> this channel is here for everyone's enjoyment, so please be nice**	*Amazing attempt to control chatters*
Dolly	> was anyone offended	*Obviously not appreciated*
XTC	> teenqueen stats	
Channel host	**> you were told to change your nickname**	
Host_sux	> is that better	*Another anti-social act*
Channel host	**> Host_sux, please change your nickname**	
Teenqueen	> why are we worried about nicknames when my best friend died last night	*Attempt to get sympathy and attention*
Dolly	> are you ok I can understand perfectly	*Attempt successful!*
Teenqueen	> how could you understand I found her dead and blue it's horrible I can't get the picture out of my mind	
RUREADY	> if your friend's just died why do you wanna chat	*Not such nice attention, but attention none the less*
Dolly	> see you	*Obviously put off by Teenqueen – will probably go to another chat room*
Host_sux	> bye every1	
Dreamboy	> don't go everyone	*Plans to stay on a lot longer*

trouble is, these young people think they are learning these skills. They believe they are not isolated and are comforted by the fact that they have many friends and an active 'social life'.

But we believe many of these young people are kidding themselves because the fact is they are isolated. Face-to-face contact is very different to staring at a computer screen. In fact, it is much harder; it takes many more skills. It takes effort, and it's better for us.

▶ Ashley's story (19 years)

Ashley looked forward to university. She worked hard, got the marks and started her uni degree. She wasn't so much looking forward to the lectures or the study. She was keen to make new friends. After the typically awkward start, the friendships were formed. It became harder to attend lectures because so much was happening on campus. Ashley turned up every day but spent most of her time having coffee with her new friends. They went out on weekends and in the term breaks. It was exactly what she had imagined and had hoped for.

This pattern went on for the entire first year. The summer holidays were busy – many friends to meet up with, to go away with. Then came second year. It started off well socially. Everyone was back in the coffee shops and in the bars. Not many lectures were attended. Because Ashley had only achieved passes in her first year, she looked around for another way to catch up on the notes she missed by not going to lectures. She found a way – the Internet. Ashley discovered that instead of relying on someone else's notes, she could download the entire lecture from the Net. Problem solved! She started socialising during the day and logging on at night. While on the Net one night she quickly emailed a uni friend to comment on the boring content of a lecture that she was printing. The friend responded almost immediately. They chatted for a while and logged off. The next night she emailed this same friend and a few more friends. They found they were able to connect with their friends at night, ▶

without having to go to the effort of using the phone.

After a few weeks of this, Ashley started really enjoying her Internet contact with her friends. She was still downloading the lectures, and she was socialising. Soon there became no need to go to uni at all. She believed she was achieving everything by staying home. The Internet chats became four and five hour marathons. She dealt with the lectures during the day and the socialising at night – all on the Net.

Passes were still achieved, but Ashley was proud of herself because she didn't even have to leave the house to pass. It took her six months to realise that most nights and every weekend were being spent on the Net. No-one was making an effort to go out any more. There wasn't any need. One minute she had felt surrounded by friends, the next completely alone. She spent the next holidays at home. When the final term of year two started, Ashley sought our help. She was depressed and slightly socially anxious. She was thinking of deferring her studies.

When she came for help, she could not believe that her use of the Internet was a problem. She only realised the significance of the problem when we addressed the depression by trying to increase her activity level. At this point Ashley found that she no longer had the confidence to meet up with people in person. The idea of ringing someone and suggesting they meet for coffee was now foreign and uncomfortable. ◄

For some parents, it may be a relief that their children are not going out all the time. Somehow the sight of a young adult at the computer is comforting – they must be working, studying hard. Many parents would presume the communication is all work-related and therefore necessary. The fact that their children are home a lot may not sound any alarm bells. But to us – the alarm bells are clanging.

These same parents will be asking their children in a couple of years: *Why aren't you in a serious relationship? Why don't you get out more? The exams are over, go out and have fun, or at least get a job.* Unfortunately, this may be the first time these parents realise their children have no longer got the confidence to go out and have fun, let alone attend a job interview.

Inappropriate online behaviour

Another problem for some teenagers is behaving online in an inappropriate manner. It's as if they tune out from the normal rules of conduct when they are in front of their computer screen, failing to see that the Internet is a part of 'real' life. Students can easily act impulsively and send out offensive emails or perpetuate hurtful rumours about students and teachers alike without thinking about the consequences. Obviously these kinds of actions aren't new and have been around in school playgrounds for years, but the mere make-up of the Internet means that such comments are more far reaching. Unfortunately, this works against some teenagers who have trouble controlling their temper and the repercussions can be great for both the sender and the receiver.

With people they don't know

Now let's look at the issues that arise when teenagers are talking online with people they have never met.

Yesterday's pen pals are today's e-pals

Remember having a pen pal when you were young? That person lived on the other side of the world and lived an incredibly different life to you. You agonisingly wrote a letter to your pen pal once or twice a year and were overjoyed when you received a letter back. You may have even dreamed of visiting your pen pal sometime. You swapped photos, but you weren't able to really know what they looked like. There was no doubt that your pen pal was a friend, but a very different friend to your real-life friends. You never put your life on hold for your pen pal, they were just a very small part of your world.

Pen pals have become e-pals. E-pals are friends who chat over the Internet. They know a lot about each other, and may even have seen a picture of one another, but until they meet face to face they do not really know each other. The problem lies in the fact that these e-pals are not just writing to each other once or twice a year. They are often talking to each other daily. And unlike having that pen pal, lives are being put on hold for e-pals. Much more time and effort goes into maintaining these relationships. That time and effort would be better spent on developing real-life friendships.

Who are they talking to?

Every parent's worst nightmare is to have their child preyed upon by a paedophile. So how do we tell teenagers that the person to whom they are chatting may not be who they think they are? As we have said, on the Internet you can say anything about yourself. Recently we went into a teenage chat room and started chatting. Before long, we were asked 'what's your a/s/l?' After asking for a translation, we were told 'a/s/l' meant age/sex/location. We felt a bit self-conscious about our real ages so we underplayed it and said we were about thirty. This got a 'lol' (laugh out loud) response from our new *friends* who quickly asked what two 30-year-olds were doing in a teenage chat room. Significantly, the chat continued. We could have been a 50-year-old paedophile for all they knew. They were willing to discuss all sorts of things, even though they knew we were not teenagers.

How do you know your teenager is not talking to a man who says he's a woman; or a woman who says she's a girl; or two men who say they are one boy? You don't – so be aware.

As with many potential dangers in life, people believe: *It will never happen to me.* They also believe they are good judges of character: *I know this person is who they say they are, I can just tell.* Teenagers particularly can be naive and often act in a way that suggests they are ignorant of these dangers. Nowhere are people more likely to be wrong when it comes to judging the trustworthiness of another human being than on the Net. As soon as you register for a chat room it asks you to pick a name. While we would discourage teenagers from using their real name, the fact that such a practice is encouraged indicates that this is not a place for complete honesty.

N E W S F L A S H

Australian police have arrested two men on child sex-related offences even though no real children were involved. Brisbane police went undercover on the Internet, posing as children to lure suspected paedophiles. The men were arrested when they arrived to rendezvous with 'children' they had met online.

The Sunday Mail 1/4/01

It's often about sex ...

In many chat rooms any comment is taken sexually. The most innocent of questions is seen as a reference to some erotic or pornographic act. Take a look at a lot of the names people give themselves – many are sexual in nature. This is harmless to a degree, but worrying to another. The sexual references are worrying because teenagers are learning and practising their flirting skills in an unnatural medium. There will never be a day when you will be able to go up to someone in person and talk in such an explicit way. If young people become comfortable talking in this way on the Net, how are they to learn the much harder skills of developing a sexual relationship with someone in real life?

In the 1980s there were safe-sex campaigns that attempted to reduce the spread of HIV and AIDS. The message was clear – you can't stop people having sex, but you can warn them of the dangers involved with unsafe sex so they can make informed choices. The same can be said of Internet usage – you can't stop teenagers using the Net but you can warn them about the many dangers, including cyber sex. Teenagers need to have available the necessary information to allow them to make informed decisions. The good news is they will not contract HIV from the Internet, but they may still be exploited and emotionally abused. Their innocence can be taken away, without them even knowing it.

In real life, we discourage teenagers from becoming sexually active too early. The reasons for this are not purely health related but emotional as well. Once a teenager becomes sexually active in one relationship, it is very hard for them not to sexualise future relationships. That is, any relationship they have from then on will probably involve sex, even if there is no sign of love or commitment. With the Internet, the same can occur, without the teenager even being aware of it. If they are having cyber sex, they are more likely to have cyber sex with others online *and* they are more likely to be sexually active in their real-life relationships.

We are giving this message to the teenagers we see, but the same message needs to be spread a lot further through books such as these, and through parents and teachers.

N E W S F L A S H

A recent report issued by the Crime Against Children Research Centre has found that 25 percent of young Americans have been exposed to pornography and 20 percent have been sexually approached.

The Sydney Morning Herald 6/00

... but not always – gore sites, hate sites

A recent conference on prejudice on the Internet highlighted the increasing amount of bigotry and hatred. So-called 'hate sites' allow people to anonymously voice their prejudices and find like-minded people. How are some of our teenagers to know that such views are not socially acceptable? They can find a lot of good and a lot of truth on the Internet, but how are they to distinguish between the right and the wrong? Without parental guidance, it makes it harder for these young people to learn.

A growing number of teenagers are also visiting sites where they can view gory pictures of people and animals. Innocent minds can be easily influenced by these images. They are probably the same sort of images parents are preventing them from watching on film. Many parents would be unaware that such sites even exist on the Internet. Then there are the sites that incite violence by, for example, showing you how to build a bomb; and cult-like sites such as suicide sites. Unfortunately, these types of sites can lead vulnerable people to make ill-informed decisions that cannot be reversed. These may sound a bit extreme to a lot of parents, but the sites exist and it is hard to know what your child is tapping into.

Global peer pressure

There has always been and will continue to be a problem with peer pressure. Teenagers want to conform, to fit in. Parents are often placed in a difficult position where they can see their child needs to fit in but are worried about the influence certain friends are having on their child.

The Internet brings a whole new dimension to the area of peer pressure. Now, not only are your children being influenced by their friends at school and down the street, they are also being influenced by teenagers and others on the other side of the world. Your child may have lived a fairly sheltered life up until now. You may hope that their experience of life will gradually grow. But with the Net, they are communicating with others who most probably have had far greater experience and therein a problem arises.

The Net is dominated by US youth culture at present. We are beginning to see the effect of information flowing across the world on our young people's minds. What is a teenager to think if all they read on the Net are stories of greater freedom and different social rules? Surely these same teenagers are going to start questioning their own parenting. Normal rebellion can become exacerbated. You may be comfortable with your child's circle of friends but do you know their Internet circle? We refer to this new form of peer pressure as *global peer pressure.* We believe it will present a new challenge for parenting in the next few years, and being forewarned is forearmed.

Unknown personalities

Another important issue is that the influence on your child may be coming from either disturbed or needy people. We are not saying that only disturbed or needy people use the Internet to meet people, but we are saying that some do. Therefore, it is highly likely that at least some of the people chatting with your child are not exerting the best influence on them. You may not be entirely happy with everyone in their real-life circle but at least you have an idea of who they are. If one of their e-pals has a very dependent personality, for example, this friend is likely to be very demanding when it comes to time spent chatting with your child. What follows is that your child may start to think that *true* friends are that close and that intense.

A more frightening example may be that one of your child's e-pals has an anti-social personality and therefore talks about activities that are anything but socially acceptable. Young people are easily impressed by such demonstrations of apparent bravery and may not be aware of the disturbed nature of some of the antics. In real life, you would be able to meet or hear about this friend and therefore have at least some idea what you're up against. On the Net, it's all done away from parental eyes but the effects are still there.

What else are teenagers doing online?

The activities of teenagers on the Net are varied. Only your teenagers can tell you what they are doing, if they want to that is. One of the most popular online pastimes is chatting via email, instant messaging, or using chat rooms. Another common activity is using bulletin boards and associated chat rooms set up around specific topics. For example, there may be a bulletin board to hear news about their favourite sporting team. Unfortunately, the bulletin board may also be set up around disturbing topics. Playing interactive games online is also popular with teenagers. They can be very addictive and adolescents can find themselves playing them for hours and hours on end. Another worrying aspect to some of the games is that there is scope within them to divulge personal information to other players, which can be dangerous. Finally, teenagers are using the Internet as a way to exchange information. They are downloading music, videos and pornography. This exchange of material can therefore be very beneficial at times, but harmful at others.

A foreign language

Go into a chat room – a teenage chat room. Read the language and try to stay calm.

 How to find a chat room

Here are some simple steps to get into a chat room to observe what goes on.

1. Log onto the Internet.

2. Find a search engine and type in the word 'chat' and click on Search.

3. Choose from the list of chat sites – start with a general one.

4. Select a specific room such as 'teenage chat'.

5. Accept the terms and conditions.

6. Either simply observe, or enter a nickname and chat (you'll probably have to ask the others online to translate some of the language).

These young people are really talking this way. The language is full of jargon and, if you do manage to understand it, is very coarse. The Net allows people to let go of their inhibitions, to drop social graces and swear and be bigots. It's as if the Net puts up a wall of sorts that allows people to be 'unseen' and unaccountable. But what gets forgotten is that the Internet is very visible and behaviour easily monitored. There are apparent rules of conduct about language and racism, but as far as we could see on many sites – these rules were ignored. It may all seem like a bit of light-hearted fun but communicating this way can easily become a habit. And if all they do is spend time in chat rooms talking in a way that is generally socially unacceptable, it will soon become harder to communicate normally when they do meet people face to face.

Teenagers have always had another language – that's healthy. But because the teenagers of the past were spending a lot of their time out in social situations, the language was restricted. Nowadays, the socialisation is mainly done in the privacy of the home and so the language is never questioned in public. Learning to behave online in a socially acceptable way is one of the greatest challenges teenagers face on the Net.

The technological generation gap

Children often know more than their parents about the latest technology. We call this the *technological generation gap*. When we were growing up we think it's fair to say that our parents knew or had experienced what we were likely to encounter as teenagers, including cigarettes, alcohol and sex. They had a sense of it and the dangers. Now, there are not that many parents of teenagers who would have a great knowledge of the Internet. Therefore it is harder for them to moderate its influence.

Often power struggles with parents that are normal through adolescence will be stronger here because of the lack of knowledge many parents have about the Internet. Because the parents are often unfamiliar with the Internet, they can become either blasé or fearful about it.

The fortunate thing about the Internet is that parents can experience some of what their children are experiencing. Indeed, we recommend that parents do log on and explore their children's favourite sites and chat rooms. Sit down with your children and ask them to show you around the Net. If your children refuse, in some cases you can use the History and Favourites icons to explore where your children have been. But sometimes this may be quite difficult or even impossible. If they have their own password, you may not be able to access where they go. Similarly, it is very easy for anyone to conceal their movements on the Internet, and this type of information is readily passed around the school playground. Being upfront with your children is really the best option.

Some parents, like Janet, have expressed concern that they would be crossing the line and invading their children's privacy if they were to do this. Obviously, this is a personal choice, and depends on the age of your children. But we think reviewing where your child has visited online is quite different from reading their private diary, for example, because the Internet is actually bringing the outside world and its dangers into your home. Furthermore the Internet infiltrates your home without your regulation or approval. Since it's an interactive communication tool, it therefore calls for greater control than your child's private thoughts recorded in their own diary. You do need to let your children know that you might access the computer occasionally.

If you know what you are dealing with, you can act appropriately. If, for example, you find that your children are merely using teenage chat rooms to talk with a few friends, and are exploring innocent sites, a gentle chat about what to watch out for would be all that was needed. If, on the other hand, you believe your children are entering into age-inappropriate chat rooms or sites, more action is needed. See the next chapter for guidelines for parents.

▶ Janet's story [45 years]

We have only been online since my oldest child became a freshman in college, one year ago. My husband and I are like 'newborn infants' when it comes to the Internet, trying to figure out what we are supposed to be doing, while our children seem to have the 'adult' role. They seemingly know how to manoeuvre their way around the www.coms, .orgs and .edus with ease. But unlike an adult their patience level with the 'infants' is very low. They explain things so quickly and in a language we do not ▶

understand. If we look puzzled for too long, they tell us to move over and they tap, tap, tap away at the keyboard and magically the information we are looking for appears before us on the screen. They then walk away shaking their heads and muttering about the incompetence that surrounds them. This is very frustrating.

My husband and I try to figure out how to find information on the Internet but find ourselves facing the possibility of downloading some dreadful virus, or receiving security violations. When we check our emails we find that quite a bit of pornography has been sent to us. We wonder how did we get on such a list. Our children tell us 'Don't open it, just delete it'. But we're still left wondering how the heck did we get on a pornographic email list?

We are aware that there is some way in which we can check to see what chat rooms and websites our children visit. But we don't know how to do this. Our friends seem to be in the same boat. We also feel a little ambivalent about checking up on our children, as they are nineteen and eighteen years old. We believe we should continue respecting their privacy but we are curious as to why we get so many pornographic emails.

Maybe some day when they are both away at college and we can use the computer without having to depend on them, we will figure out what to do! Then we might be able to find out which chat rooms and websites the kids visited and the answer to our question! ◄

General effects

Some general psychological effects of teenagers spending too much time online are listed below. These effects can be clustered into a couple of groups. First there is the effect of a limited social life, and the social isolation and possible anxiety and depression that follow decreasing levels of confidence. Second there are the dangers of peer pressure from different cultures and the increased likelihood that they will be exposed to inappropriate material on the Net. Parents need to be aware of these effects because the teenagers are most probably blissfully ignorant.

Effects of too much time on the Net

- limits social circle to those online
- decreases confidence in face-to-face contact
- social isolation – which can lead to increased anxiety and increased depression
- physical inactivity – which can lead to both emotional and physical problems such as depression and obesity
- reduced incentive to make any effort to see people
- peer pressure from all around the world – *global peer pressure*
- increased likelihood of exposure to inappropriate material on the Net

Jealousy

An unexpected problem of chat room use is jealousy. We have seen many people, not just teenagers, who become jealous of practical strangers on the Net. Jealousy happens when two people become friends on the Net; perhaps they chat daily to each other. One day, one of the friends may 'catch' the other talking to a third person, or a fourth person. When they announce that they are now online, they expect their friend to cease talking to the others. If this doesn't happen, jealousy can creep in.

In other cases, three or four e-pals may be regular chatters. These friends may be at different parts of the globe – thus necessitating careful planning to accommodate the different time zones. If one of the friends is not present at a chat session, jealousy can once again set in. They can feel left out, isolated, and even anxious or depressed. Such jealousy is often present in real-life friendships, but it seems to be a particular problem in Internet friendships. Many people go to the length of leaving their computers logged on so they can be 'beeped' whenever their friends are online. You can imagine the time and money this takes.

School or university friends who also go online to chat can become jealous of the time one person spends chatting to another. In this way, there is an extension of the normal jealousy in teen relationships being carried over from school to the Net at night.

As is always the case, jealousy is a very unhealthy emotion and can lead to problems with anxiety and/or depression. In order to eliminate jealousy, the thoughts that lead to the emotion need to be challenged. For example, when their friend is caught chatting to someone else, the teenager may think:

> *They don't like me. They're organising to meet without me. There must be something wrong with me.*

As we have outlined in the section on clear thinking in Chapter 9, we would encourage someone thinking this way, to ask themselves:

> *Where is the evidence they don't like me or there's something wrong with me?*

> *What are the consequences of thinking this way?*

> *How would I advise a friend who was thinking this way?*

By asking themselves these questions, they may be able to think in a more healthy way such as:

> *Just because they're chatting without me, doesn't mean they don't like me, or that there's something wrong with me. Perhaps they found each other online by accident, or perhaps that was a more suitable time to talk. I will chat with them when I can, but also chat with others as well as catching up with my real-life friends.*

By thinking in this more helpful way, jealousy can be reduced and hopefully eliminated.

Now we've identified the problems for teens, it's really important for parents to know what steps they can take to help guide and protect their children online. In the next chapter we outline our advice to help keep your children on the right side of the Net.

In brief...

- Too much time on the Internet has its consequences.
- Chat room talk is an entirely different language.
- Teenagers are exposed to **global peer pressure** via the Net.
- There is a **technological generation gap** in many families.

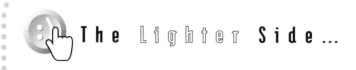

The Lighter Side ...

Irish virus

Received by email:

Top of the mornin' to ya.

I'm an Irish virus and I'll be needing your help to spread. Please copy me and forward me to everyone in your personal address book there.

Tanks very much.

* * *

Funny definitions

MOUSE POTATO: The online, wired generation's answer to the couch potato.

PERCUSSIVE MAINTENANCE: The fine art of whacking the heck out of an electronic device to get it to work again.

VULCAN NERVE PINCH: The taxing hand position required to reach all the appropriate keys for certain commands. For instance, rebooting a Mac II computer involves simultaneously pressing the Control key, the Command key, the Return key, and the Power On key.

404: Someone who's clueless. From the World Wide Web error message '404 Not Found,' meaning that the requested document could not be located.

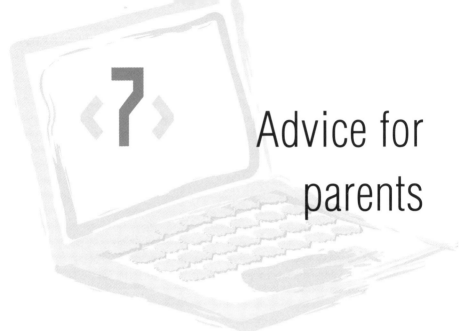

< 7 > Advice for parents

Now we have outlined some of the problems teenagers face when using the Internet, we would like to give you some guidelines for managing these issues. As is always the case, you'll need to tailor our ideas to fit in with your family's values and beliefs. We want to give you a starting point so you may know where to go from here.

What should parents do?

We are often asked by parents: *How do we stop our children from getting into trouble on the Internet?* At the end of the day, nothing is foolproof. There are no guarantees. But we strongly believe you can put safeguards in place to help your children make decisions that are in their best interest.

We encourage parents to talk to their children about how they spend their time on the Internet, and to learn about the Internet by reading about it or taking a course. Our motto to any parent is: ***Get informed and take action.*** So, the next time your child is surfing the Net, sit with them and ask them to show you what they do. Ask them to take you into a chat room. If you've never been in one, it'll be an interesting experience. As we have said, you'll have to get your child to decipher the jargon as you go.

We're not suggesting you race off to university and obtain a degree in computer science but we do believe there are many steps you can take to help protect your kids online.

It's important that your children learn how valuable the Internet is as an educational resource as well as being aware of its downside. We think it's really important for parents to show children how to use the Internet in an appropriate way. The following exercise will help you do this.

How to make the Internet a valuable learning experience for your child

- Set a regular time on a weekly basis for you and your child to explore the Internet. This way your child looks forward to the activity and can think about it in advance.

- Find out what are good sites for you and your child to visit. Make a list of their favourite ones that you can then pass onto other parents. If you don't know where to begin, ask your child's school to recommend some, check your local library, ask other parents, or buy a book that lists fun sites to visit with children.

- Encourage your child to offer suggestions, and then together you can check out the appropriateness of the site.

- If you encounter a site that you think isn't appropriate, show your child why so they understand, then look together for a more suitable one.

- Encourage your children to think critically about the information they view. Do they agree with everything they see? How can they check the facts? Is the site trying to promote a certain product?

- Make the experience an enjoyable one.

- Include younger children when appropriate.

If you do not think your teenager has a problem

Many parents will be interested in reading about the issues associated with teenage Internet use, but do not believe their child has a problem. We would still encourage these parents to get informed. The old adage 'prevention is better than cure' is useful in this context.

Get informed

We believe that in life, knowledge is power. Blissful ignorance can be dangerous – especially when it comes to what goes on on the Net. We are all on a very steep learning curve; the ethical and legal guidelines regarding the Internet's use are continually evolving but remain a few steps behind the users and abusers of the Internet. The following table may give you some ideas about how to get informed.

 Ways to get informed

- Attend a course, e.g. adult education classes.
- Visit the library and borrow an introductory book on the Internet.
- Contact your child's school and find out what they are teaching about all aspects of the Internet, particularly about safety and acceptable use.
- Suggest to your child's school that they have a seminar for parents on what their children are learning.
- Ask your child what they are learning.
- Ask your child to show you what they do online, which websites they like to visit and which chat rooms they use.
- Talk to other parents – what limits do they set?
- Be aware of the danger signs for Internet addiction in teenagers (see Chapter 6).

Take action

After you've learnt more about the Internet and what your child may be doing, it's a good idea to become involved. Keep the computer out of their bedroom. If your child is using the computer to study and therefore needs peace and quiet, try and keep the noise level down. Maybe you need to turn the TV off or remove other children to different areas of the house. Whatever the case, stay in touch with your child while they are online.

Every now and then, stop and look at the screen and ask them to show you around the Net or the chat room they are using. Show mild interest and then move on. Again the message is clear – anything you are doing should be all right for a parent to watch (if only for a minute). If your child types 'pos', be warned, as that stands for 'parent over shoulder'. You may need to investigate further.

One word of advice: try not to show shock when you see some of the language used and the content of some of the conversations. Instead, try to talk openly with your child about the Internet. If you're worried about something you see, calmly discuss your concern with them. Talk about the positives and the negatives. You want the message they take away to be that you are willing and available to discuss anything that comes up on the Net, no matter how perverted or horrible. You need to be sure they understand that people can be whoever they like online, and that most people lie about some aspect of themselves when online.

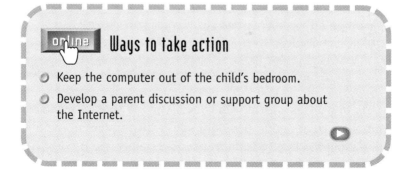

online   Ways to take action

- Keep the computer out of the child's bedroom.
- Develop a parent discussion or support group about the Internet.

- Discuss family values and beliefs with your children.
- Act as a parental team when you talk with your children.
- Be consistent across family with limits on Internet use.
- Go into chat rooms with your children from time to time.
- Model to your children how to use the Internet appropriately to gain information.
- Encourage them to tell you if they are uncomfortable.
- Bridge the technology gap between you and your child.
- Find out what rules your children's friends' parents set.

 Katie.com

Katie.com is a must-read for all parents with children who use the Internet. Katie tells her story of how in 1995 she became inadvertently involved with a paedophile on the Internet. She was thirteen years old at the time and lived in Connecticut, US. What started out for Katie as friendship and someone to confide in, ended in a meeting approximately six months later with the guy she thought was her boyfriend. He ended up being a paedophile, some twenty years older than he told her, who assaulted her. Katie gives her readers a good insight into how a paedophile preys on his innocent victims and how the latter are helpless to protect themselves.

Try to work as a team with your partner. If you are separated from your child's other parent, it still helps to present a united front about the Internet and its use. It certainly doesn't work if a child has unlimited access in one house and not in the other.

Family values and beliefs

◉ What values and beliefs do you hold as a family?

From an early age, start discussing with your children the values and beliefs that are important in your home and within your society. For example, you may discuss the normal rules of your house, such as respecting each other's wishes and talking in a polite manner. Having a framework like this makes it much easier when talking about what behaviour is appropriate on the Net and what isn't – you are telling them that the same rules apply. It is also useful to introduce your teenager to the possibility that from time to time they'll encounter people or information on the Net that doesn't fit with the values and beliefs of your family. They then need to know what they should do in such a situation.

 What your children should tell themselves

◉ This person or site does not match my family's values and beliefs.

◉ I should stop talking to this person.

◉ I should tell my parents.

◉ I should think about letting the chat room host know if the information is highly inappropriate to a teenage chat room.

Set some limits

You also need to decide what limits you want to put in place. Do you wish to use blocks that prevent access to certain websites such as those with adult pornography or hate sites? (Be warned: these programs aren't foolproof.) How long will you allow your child to be online? When? How does homework fit in? Will you allow them to buy any products online? Limits should be placed on time, topic and task. That is, it should be clear to any child how long they are allowed to be online, what sites they can visit and which tasks they are permitted to perform (for example, games, email, chat).

▶ Emily's story [43 years]

Four years ago, when my eldest son was seven, the Internet was not yet a big thing in America. But my son already knew his way around a computer. When I'd occasionally walk into the office to see what he was doing, he would tell me he was just playing a game or sorting out cards. To me he looked nervous as though he had something to hide.

At about the same time I learnt from friends that you could find out what sites had been visited on a computer by using the History button, so that's what we did. My hunch was right. My son had typed in the word 'sex' that had led him to many different sites. No wonder he often looked like he'd been caught doing something he shouldn't have been.

In the end, it wasn't the fact that he was interested in sex that was the problem because that's a normal part of growing up, but it was the lying that bothered me. He knew he was being deceptive. We addressed the lying and I explained to him that there are some people out there who are interested in kids for unsavoury purposes. After that incident he was not allowed to surf the web without our permission.

With our younger children it hasn't really been an issue because we are a little wiser. They spend most of their time playing interactive games with their friends. We don't use blocks, probably more out of laziness than anything else, but we are very open with them about the dangers of the Internet. If however, for example, they are younger than the recommended minimum age to play a game, we tell them that they have to stick by the rules because they have been set for a reason.

Overall our general rule is that irrespective of whether it is television, game boys, computer games or the Internet, they aren't allowed to use any of them until all of their homework and music practice is complete. They seem to accept this. ◀

Emily's story reminds us that as parents you need to become informed. She followed the advice from friends to use the History icon to explore where her son had been on the Internet. Once again, we need to warn you that children and adolescents can quite quickly learn how to cover their tracks on the Net, so don't allow yourself to be lulled into a false sense of security when there is no evidence of them visiting inappropriate sites. Our message is a consistent one – the most important strategy any parent can use is to teach their children about appropriate behaviour on and off the Net. Relying on History or Favourites icons, or software filtering programs, will not protect your children from harm.

N E W S F L A S H

An Australian Information Technology company has developed a product that can be bought by the parents of latchkey children. The service uses web cams in the house so that working parents can semi-supervise their kids when they get home from school.

The Sydney Morning Herald 15/3/01

If your child isn't doing anything to harm themselves or others (such as clocking up huge bills on the Net by shopping or gambling; abusing people; or visiting pornographic, gore or hate sites) you may need to let go and let them make their own choices. As long as you've been clear and open about your concerns, all you can do is hope that your words will influence the choices they make at some stage. Don't fall into the trap of thinking that by simply limiting their access you've solved the problem. Remember, they can always go somewhere else. It is far easier to keep an eye on your children if they use the Internet at home rather than at a friend's house. The same rules that apply to experimenting with alcohol and sex apply to Internet use.

T

▶ **Winnie's story [44 years]**

My son is now twenty and my daughter fifteen. There's just the three of us. We've had access to the Internet from home for only about three years now, partly because getting set up is expensive and also because I was a bit worried about the dangers of cyberspace psychos ... but I guess they're everywhere, aren't they?

My son, who is at college, is an extreme extrovert and he uses it very little. I think he uses it for paying bills, and occasionally to read the news and surf around. But he has much more of an affinity for the telephone and voice mail! My daughter on the other hand uses the Internet every day. She talks to friends quite a lot and seeks out particular websites as she has a strong interest in marine biology.

When we first connected to the Internet I was concerned to protect my then twelve-year-old. Our service provider offered what seemed like protected access so we chose them. I also decided to put the computer desk in the 'heart' of the house, where there was lots of traffic and people cooking, eating, doing dishes and laundry, talking on the phone and watching television. This allowed me to be very 'stealthy' in my supervisory capacity, without obviously peering over her shoulder to see the screen. Both of those strategies have been successful.

It seems as though my concerns for my daughter about the potential abuses of the Internet have pretty much faded. This could be a function of her particular temperament and personality. The most challenging thing I've had to manage is the amount of time 'wasted' talking to friends from school when homework should be getting done. Since my daughter is relatively 'school smart' and performs at a high level, she's pretty self-motivated and I typically only issue a stern reminder and that's it.

I suspect, however, that some parents think that when their kids are online they're not hassling anybody, they're quiet, and it can seem like they're engaged in something appropriate. Meanwhile advertisers are potentially winning their minds and hearts! I personally think this is more of a problem than their ⏵

vulnerability to predators, or access to dangerous information such as how-to-make-a-bomb.

I guess for me, I think it falls into the category of media literacy. The world our kids are going into is moving faster and faster all the time. The Internet is here to stay and it has been thoroughly integrated into their culture. Kids need to be able to manage it in their lives, to use it as an appropriate tool, to understand its benefits and to think critically about its abuses. Like television, radio, video, movies and mobile phones, they need to know when to turn it off and to consider the source. In a democracy like America it is vital for citizens to think critically about everything. We need to equip kids more in terms of their inner stuff ... the 'universe behind their eyes' ... then they will be free enough and smart enough to manage the Internet or whatever all else comes their way. ◀

Limits can be set using ground rules, especially about what information they give to their online friends. Then children know where they stand and there shouldn't be any doubt about where you draw the line. As is nearly always the case with parenting, children benefit from limits being placed on them.

 Some ground rules

It is recommended that children:

- never give their real name to anyone online, nor other personal information, such as their school, what activities they do, or where they live – teach them to be evasive and to proceed with caution
- never meet anyone they have met online
- never email their picture to anyone
- tell you if they want to talk on the telephone with someone they have met online – if you can, discourage this ▶

but at least then you have the opportunity to monitor the call; use a block of your telephone number before the call is made

- do not send out derogatory emails about any person
- try to avoid being a part of the Internet rumour mill

Teaching your children to be evasive may feel as though you are encouraging them to lie. We believe, however, that teenagers need to be evasive online to protect themselves. There are warning messages that flash across the screens of teenage chat rooms. They say: *Don't give out personal information while chatting. Protect yourself from Internet abuse.* If your children are reading this message and hearing it from their parents, they may start listening. Teaching them the difference between being cautious and lying is a valuable lesson. It's good to go that one step further and teach children how to respond assertively to people asking them for personal details:

I'm not allowed to give out my name, address, phone number or photo to people my parents haven't spoken to or met.

 ## Teach your children to behave assertively

What is assertiveness?
Simply, it is telling the truth in an appropriate manner.

Why is it important?
To enable you to behave in a way that does not compromise your standards or values.

How do I teach them?
Explain what assertiveness means, why it is important and how you can feel used if you don't stand up for yourself.

Use examples that are appropriate for their age, making sure to teach them to use the word 'I' in the responses they give. For example: *No thanks; I don't want to give you that information.* Role model different situations with them – they don't have to be Internet-related situations.

▶ Advice from a school superintendent about the Internet

First and foremost, I believe that when used appropriately, the Internet is a powerful educational tool. We [in the US] are only just beginning to understand how it can enhance and improve learning opportunities for our students. However, we are also discovering many issues that arise with students on the Internet. We need to be working with parents to address these problems.

I think the biggest challenge teachers and parents face is educating children about appropriate behaviour on the Internet. Many children don't think the Internet is a part of 'real' life and often their behaviour reflects this. For example, a student who would know it's unacceptable to open someone else's regular mail may not have a second thought about attempting to outsmart the computer system to gain access to another person's email account. They need to learn that the Internet is a part of 'real' life and the same rules of appropriate behaviour apply.

The types of Internet related problems that teachers have to manage in schools today tend to fall into two main categories. The first category involves dealing with students who make serious errors of judgement on the Internet. Such errors of judgement include sending derogatory emails to students or teachers, accessing inappropriate information on the Internet, passing on to other students information about inappropriate sites, perpetuating rumours by email and instant messaging, violating another person's privacy online and wasting too much valuable time. The second category includes managing potential crises where safety issues are crucial. In these cases information is communicated via the Internet that may suggest that a person's safety is at risk. ◉

It is important to remember, however, that these behaviours also occur outside the Internet. As there is only so much anyone can control, teachers and parents alike need to encourage appropriate online behaviour. ◄

We are grateful to have been able to include this helpful advice to parents from a school superintendent. It is up to parents to protect their children from the dangers of the Internet because the activity is most often taking place outside school hours. Schools can attempt to educate and regulate, but without the involvement of the parents, children can be at risk.

As the superintendent said, inappropriate behaviour also occurs outside the Internet. That is, the behaviour itself is not new, just the way it is carried out. For example, the schoolyard bully has always existed, but with the Internet this bullying behaviour can have disastrous consequences if the teasing and harassment is carried out on a large scale via the Net. Just as the victim of the schoolyard bully may not speak up to their parents because of shame, embarrassment or fear, a victim of Internet bullying or harassment may not inform their parents. Parents need to be aware that problems such as this exist and be on the lookout for signs that their child may be experiencing difficulties. By encouraging them to talk to you about anything they see on the Net that disturbs them, you may make it easier for your child to speak up.

► Issues about students and the Internet

As a high school teacher of personal development [in Australia], I think some important issues with students and the Internet are:

1. Schools need to be committed to training staff in advanced technology and keeping up to date with current developments as teenagers are streets ahead of parents and teachers about the Internet.

2. Ensure school students are taught accurate research skills, the correct way to acknowledge sources of information and the dangers of plagiarism, as downloading masses of information is appealing for tasks, but dangerous if overused.

3. Many children are spending in excess of six hours nightly 'surfing the Net', emailing and accessing chat rooms, which can have many negative effects. Therefore parental supervision of time spent on the computer at home and sites visited is essential. Too many children are accessing age-inappropriate sites and this needs to be carefully monitored.

4. Teenagers are learning to use informal written language that does not always 'translate' or convey the spoken message. Innuendo and misunderstandings frequently occur because of misinterpretation.

5. Many homes only have one computer yet several school-aged children are expected to complete homework and assignments. Competition for access time can result in nightly disharmony in the home, and late homework for school.

6. Some young students have difficulty putting pen to paper and have to relearn basic coordination skills, which have been neglected after years of typing. Others have begun to notice neck and back pain or discomfort because they are either not taught or are not practising correct posture or exercise necessary when spending time in one position. ◀

Remind them of their life offline

Regularly encourage your children to maintain their real-life friendships. Even if they are chatting to their school friends online, they also need to be hanging out with their friends learning how to socialise. Remember Ashley from the previous chapter? She forgot how to socialise even though she was spending four and five hours a night on the Net talking with her university friends.

Their offline life should also involve more active outdoor play that allows them just to be kids or teenagers. By using their imagination, playing a team sport and negotiating with their friends, children learn a lot about life itself. Unfortunately, overuse of the Internet is adding to the ever-increasing problem of ourselves and our children becoming sedentary and overweight.

Let's look at a case where a young woman was using the Net to avoid people.

▶ Anna's story (18 years)

Anna had been socially anxious and depressed. Her family had been very involved in her treatment and was keen to help in any way they could. Anna's parents contacted us after she had been released from hospital following a suicidal episode. Anna herself was motivated to work on her issues. She attended appointments, did homework that was set, and was generally motivated to change. All was going well until Anna found the Internet. The family got connected and she went surfing one night out of curiosity – all innocent enough, until she found the chat rooms. When online, Anna found that she was not anxious. She could open up and discuss very intimate details of her life to her chat room friends. Some people may wonder what is wrong with this. One minor problem was that Anna confessed that she sometimes pretended to be someone she wasn't – either older, from another country, or even saying she was male.

The major problem as far as we were concerned was the fact that Anna no longer thought she needed to do any of the activities she had been doing as part of the treatment for her depression and anxiety. Her needs were being met in the chat rooms and her feelings of isolation, inadequacy and generalised anxiety were not there. Her family also thought she was much improved. We had to burst this bubble. When Anna was asked how she felt about being out in public or attempting to get a part-time job, the anxiety returned with a vengeance. It became clear to Anna and her family that the problems had not been resolved, just ignored. ◀

We are not saying that anyone who uses chat rooms is depressed or socially anxious. Rather, we are saying that many individuals fail to face up to the real world because they have their needs met by the Net. Like so many things in life, balance is needed – nothing will ever replace face-to-face contact.

If you believe your teenager has a problem

First you need to learn the danger signs of Internet addiction in teenagers. Dr Kimberly Young has identified a number of signs to look out for, the presence of three or more of which might indicate Internet addiction or some other form of substance abuse. The signs are:

- excessive fatigue
- academic problems
- withdrawing from friends
- a loss of interest in other activities they have previously enjoyed
- acting out

If you think your child shows some or all of these signs, you need to take action. First, consider what else might be going on for them. Could they be taking drugs or abusing alcohol? Are they depressed or socially anxious, and perhaps using the Internet to improve the way they feel? You will need to talk to your child about your concerns. It's best if both parents can be involved in this discussion. If you believe the Internet is the problem, tell them you want to help because you are concerned about their Internet use. Try to keep it non-threatening and stick to the facts that you've observed. For example, you might say: *We're really worried about the way you're using the Internet. You're up a lot at night, you're tired, and you've been missing school. How about the three of us sit down and work out what we need to do? What do you think?*

Then you will need to set limits on their Internet use. Obviously some drastic steps, such as supervising usage, moving the computer and limiting access, may be needed. Depending on how your child accepts these limits, it may be necessary to meet with the school counsellor and seek their ideas so you can continue with the team approach. You may need to seek professional help with someone who is familiar with Internet problems. Ask your child to go along with you. If they refuse, go alone.

It may help you to ask yourself: *If I were concerned that my son or daughter had a major drug problem, how would I approach it?*

Excessive Internet use is no different. Don't believe that because they're home they must be okay.

Some common concerns

Here are some questions parents often ask us about their teenagers and the Internet.

How old should my child be to be using the Net?

If your child is over sixteen, the limits you set will be different from those you may set a twelve year-old. We would recommend that you don't allow your child unsupervised access to the Internet until they are old enough and mature enough to understand the potential problems and the consequences of their actions. Their personality and how likely you believe they would be able to set their own limits will help you to determine the limits you set. It may help to think of the limits you set with television and movies.

How long should children be on the Internet?

We'd encourage you to think how you would answer that question if you were asking it about TV use? We saw an interesting survey recently that asked teenagers who were learning about safety on the Net, how long kids should be allowed online – and their answer was 1.5 hours per day of surfing. They did say that they would need a longer amount of time if they were doing a specific assignment. This seems to be a good guideline.

What about interactive games?

Well, the same idea applies here. You have to set limits for 'game' time. We'd recommend that you actually set 'screen' time limits that include everything they do from television, to game boys, to using the Internet for surfing, games and chatting.

What if my child won't talk to me about their Internet use?

If your child will not discuss the issue of Internet use, you might conclude that there is some sort of problem that they're hiding. Emphasise your concern and your desire to work with them on the issue. Enlist the help of teachers and other parents to support the limits you have put in place. Pick your time and place to discuss the issue, and try not to attack. Once again, think about how you would address another delicate issue such as sex or drug use.

What should I do about different aged children on the Net?
You need to be very clear that different aged children need different limits for time spent online, the activities they want to partake in and the level of supervision required. Enforce the age limits set by specific websites. You need to talk to your older children about being responsible when their younger siblings are around and make sure that any Internet use mirrors the age of the youngest user.

How candid should I be about the dangers of the Internet?
Our advice is to always be honest in what you say. Your delivery of this information will, however, vary according to the age of your children. Treat it a bit like sex education – answer their questions and give accurate information for their age. Remind them to tell you about anything that worries them.

How do I work out which guidelines to use?
We recommend you involve your children in establishing computer or Internet rules. Depending on their ages, you will set different rules. You need to consider time online, the activities your children do online, and when their homework will be done. One rule of thumb is to remember that no matter what blocks or screening devices you use, information can still be accessed; nothing replaces parental supervision. Restricting general surfing is a good guideline for children younger than sixteen years of age unless there's adult supervision. If you don't really have many ideas, talk to your friends, or ask what the school recommends.

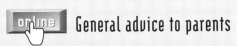

online **General advice to parents**

1. Get informed, take action.
2. Know the danger signs of Internet addiction for children (and for adults).

3. Find out what the school is teaching and what other parents are doing.
4. Learn about the Internet yourself – you're never too old.
5. Don't be lulled into a false sense of security that your children are safe because they are at home on their computer.
6. Encourage them to maintain their real-life friendships and activities.
7. Keep the computer out of the bedroom.
8. Don't be scared of the Internet.
9. Set limits – just as you've done for TV and computer games – and stick to them.
10. Supervise young children on the Net – don't see it as a babysitter.
11. Don't let children or young teenagers surf the Net without your permission.
12. Don't rely solely on filtering software to block certain sites.

At the end of the day, as your children grow up they have to make their own choices. However, as with any other behaviour, a lot of what you lay down in the formative years influences the decisions they make at some stage. The Internet will most likely change your life; it will definitely change your children's. So if you haven't already, start bridging the technological gap between you and them.

In brief...

- The Internet can be a valuable learning experience for your child.
- Get informed and take action, for the sake of your children.
- Talk to them about your family's values and beliefs.
- Set limits and ground rules for Internet use.
- Remind your children of their life offline.
- Recognise the danger signs of Internet addiction.

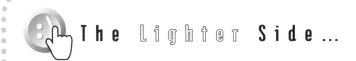

The Lighter Side...

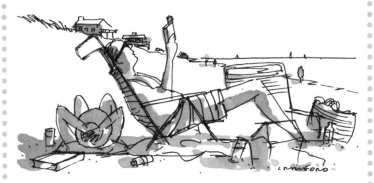

"I think I'll head back to the house for a little Net-sex and a nap."

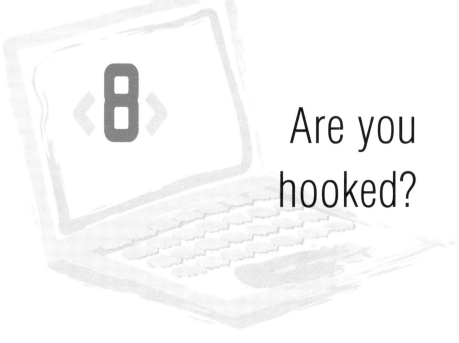

Are you hooked?

O bviously, there are many of you who have benefited from the Internet, and that's great. But now we want to turn your attention to the warning signs of excessive Internet use. Like any problem, the sooner you start doing something about it, the greater the chance of getting it under control.

Attractive yet potentially dangerous

Curiosity certainly accounts for why many people initially surf the Net. There is definitely a novelty factor. You may go online looking for something specific only to be sidetracked by something else that interests you. If you go online to chat, you can talk to many different people, be whoever you like, say whatever you like and feel somewhat smug in the process. Being anonymous makes some people feel much more confident in how they express themselves. For others it allows them to take risks they would never have dreamed of in real life. Like any activity that can become addictive, the Internet is stimulating and people feel good when they use it – well at least in the beginning.

But some of you might feel the Internet is becoming a problem for you. Do you often find yourself thinking about when you next will be able to go online? Do you think you would react negatively if your Internet connection was down for a day? Have you repeatedly gone online at work for extended periods of time for your own purposes? These questions and others like them are important because they indicate how dependent you might be on the Internet. Most people who believe they use the Internet to excess say they feel somewhat 'out of control', and that they have tried on many occasions to cut back their Internet use without any luck. Their repeated Internet use also has a negative effect on their personal, family or work life.

If you have a problem with the Internet, it most likely will be your partner, your colleague or a close friend who first expresses concern. Some of you will want to deny the problem while others will feel relieved that the topic is out in the open. Nonetheless, admitting the problem is the first step.

N E W S F L A S H

An e-store has been set up to sell the personal items of serial killers, including hair, letters, autographs and artwork. Victims' families have expressed shock and disgust.

The Sydney Morning Herald 6/00

Do you have a problem?

You may not think your Internet use is particularly a problem. Maybe if you're honest with yourself you think that sometimes you stay online a little longer than intended but believe that if you wanted to you could easily stop. Before we go any further ask yourself the questions below. If you answer 'yes' to any of these questions, the Internet may be a problem for you.

Is the Internet affecting your life?

- Has your partner complained recently about your use of the Internet?
- Have you missed or nearly missed an important appointment because of your use of the Internet?
- Have you rearranged your schedule in any way to get online?
- Have you altered your sleeping patterns to use the Internet?
- Have you overslept for work or school because of your late hours on the Net?
- Have you said you'll get off the computer, only to find yourself still online some time later?
- If you're single, how many times have you declined an invitation to go out so you could go online?
- Have you secretly gone online at work for extended periods of time for your own use?
- Has your boss complained about your work performance?

You will see that we mention going online during work hours for your own use. While most people might occasionally do this, in much the same way as you'd make the odd personal telephone call, it becomes a problem if you are doing this when it is either against your company policy or your job performance is suffering. We would be particularly concerned if you felt that you had little control over your behaviour, but continued regardless.

Some of you will categorically deny the Internet is affecting your life – even if you're on the Net for many hours a day. Although hours do not necessarily correlate with dependency, we believe that if anybody is on the Net for more than three hours per day on a regular basis (not including work or study time), they could have a problem. This figure is only a guideline but a good one. Now we'll tell you how we arrived at the magical number of three.

There are 24 hours in a day. If you sleep for eight hours on average and go to work for another eight to ten, that only leaves about six hours for all the other things you need to do in your day. If you've got a partner, children, extended family, friends and outside interests then maintaining those relationships and interests easily accounts for the remaining six hours, not to mention housework or exercise. For those of you who work inside the home, running a household and raising a family is a full-time job anyway. But the bottom line is: while you are on the Net, something else in your life is not being done because the Internet is a relatively exclusive pursuit. Even the television allows more family interaction than the Internet because you can all be watching the same program and talking about it. If you're still not convinced think about someone who uses the gym for more than three hours each day, every day. Wouldn't you think they were a little obsessed?

Hand in hand with our magical number of three is how strong your desire or urge is to log on each day. Would it worry you if for some reason you could not go online for a period of time? Have a look now at the warning signs that the Internet is becoming a problem.

online Warning signs that the Internet may be a problem for you

- You spend a lot of time thinking about your Internet activity.
- You feel a need to log on each day for long periods of time.
- Someone close to you has expressed their concern about you and the Internet.
- You have tried unsuccessfully to cut down your Internet use.
- You are eager to contact certain people online.
- You feel jealous or 'left out' if you can't join your e-friends online.

- You have attempted to contact the people you have met online in 'real' life, e.g. by telephone.
- You frequently fantasise or masturbate while online.
- You lie to your family or friends about what you do online and for how long.
- Your Internet behaviour has affected your relationships and/or your work.
- You have run up excessive bills by online shopping or Internet use.
- You repeatedly access the Internet at work for your own personal use.
- You have done something online that you regret because it contradicts your moral code.

Obviously, the more of these warning signs that you said 'yes' to, the more likely it is your Internet use is a real problem in your life. Some of you may already realise that you can no longer go on without help. Maybe you are at the point where you can see clearly that the short-term pleasure of being on the Net loses out to the long-term pain every time. Both Martha and John certainly felt this way when they finally came for help. Their stories are very different but hopefully they give you a little more insight into the potential problems associated with excessive Internet use.

▶ Martha's story (42 years)

I have been married for seventeen years. Our marriage has had its ups and downs like everybody else, but after the birth of our second child six years ago we seemed to stop talking to one another.

I started visiting chat rooms and found that I had a lot in common with some of the women I met. Most of them lived in the US. I was never interested in talking to men. I didn't want an affair. I wanted women who understood me and what I was going through. I found that just by offloading to my Internet friends, I didn't need to confront my husband about anything. Things became a lot more peaceful.

Since I had a busy full-time job, the best time for me to chat to my e-pals was in the early hours of the morning. I started setting my alarm for 3 a.m. This way, I was not disturbing anyone else, and was not taking time away from the family. I did, however, have to start going to bed fairly early to be able to function at work.

After a couple of months, my husband started complaining about the time I spent on the Net. He said I was distant and withdrawn. I guess I was to an extent, but I thought I was happy. He wanted me to talk to him about the things I talked to my e-pals about. I just couldn't. It was private. I started realising that I was getting most of my needs met from these strangers who I considered to be my closest friends in the world. Our relationship began to unravel. We stopped having sex. We no longer went out. I never saw any of my real friends any more. I was obsessed with getting to bed early so that I could wake at 3 a.m. and resume my conversations. There was no doubt I was hooked. Losing my friends and nearly losing my marriage did not prompt me to seek help though. It was when I became angry and jealous that I finally sought counselling. I had never felt jealous in my life before, but suddenly I wanted to know which of my e-pals were talking to whom and when. If I found out that two of them had chatted without me, I was overwhelmed with jealousy. I became aggressive towards them in my emails. I accused them of leaving me out and of not being 'true' friends. I could not function.

I can now see that I had been in trouble for a while. I hadn't realised the slow addiction to these chat rooms. I had talked myself into believing that these friends were more real, more important, than my marriage, children and friends. I am now working on the problem in counselling. ◄

▶ **John's story [39 years]**

John could hardly sit still. He looked tired and drawn as he talked about his predicament. He had recently separated from his wife and three children. At first he was ashamed to reveal his activities on the Internet. But after our first session he said he felt a great sense of relief to be finally talking to someone.

I feel completely out of control. I'm on the Net all night. I'm rarely in bed before 2 a.m. and then I can hardly get up in the morning for work. My life is totally stuffed. My marriage is over, I miss my kids, I'm concerned about my job, and now I'm hooked on the Internet. I spend all night on porn sites and having cyber sex with women I meet online. I hate what this is doing to me but I can't stop. I have tried many times to quit, and each time I say 'not tonight', I find myself back online before you know it.

I'm keen on a woman I've met at work and we've started seeing each other. I'm afraid that I will screw up this relationship too. Even though she's great, I'm scared to get too close. It's actually easier to meet people online and have a fling than have to worry too much about all the emotional stuff that goes with a new relationship. All I know is that I have to do something now. ◀

John was desperate; he was depressed and dependent on the Internet. He hated going online each night but couldn't stop himself. He certainly believed that the adult sites he visited were like a drug, they were too hard to resist. We are seeing more and more people like John. The Internet provides people who are experiencing difficulties in their life easy access to others who may listen to them, or easy access to some kind of activity that takes their mind off their problems. Unfortunately, many people who become dependent on the Internet already suffer from some kind of psychological problem such as depression, anxiety or chronically low self-esteem. They may also be struggling with alcohol or drug abuse. Becoming hooked on the Internet exacerbates their situation and brings on more difficulties.

What are you avoiding?

We have observed from our work that some people who get into trouble on the Internet are using it as a way of avoiding something in their life that they are finding hard to manage. In the table below we have listed Dr Kimberly Young's top ten avoidances from her research in the US. Certainly from our experience we would agree with Dr Young's findings.

 What are people avoiding? Top-ten list of avoidances

1. loneliness
2. marital discontent
3. work-related stress
4. boredom
5. depression
6. financial problems
7. insecurity about physical appearance
8. anxiety
9. struggles with recovery from other addictions
10. limited social life

When you look down this list, it's not surprising really that the Internet can help people escape from the other problems in their life. Pre-Internet it would have been harder for say someone who was depressed to become dependent on some other activity. With depression, loss of motivation and social withdrawal are central features. Where the Internet is different is that first of all you don't have to get dressed to go online; you don't even have to leave your bed. Not much effort is required, and this we believe is crucial to excessive Internet use.

It often seems that people who are unhappy about something in their lives find the Internet to be uplifting. Going online certainly helps them take their mind off the other problems they are facing. By logging on each day they avoid having to think about the other issues in their life, which immediately gives them short-term relief. Because they feel 'better' after logging on each day, they are more likely to log on the next time they are feeling down. And so the process takes on a life of its own. Before long the negative effects start to emerge.

One of the first clients we saw with an Internet problem came because she was unhappy in her marriage. She had been married for ten years and had three young children. She felt her life was passing her by and that she had achieved 'nothing'. She felt neglected by her husband who was busy pursuing his career. She missed her job too but decided to be a stay-at-home mum for the time being. After her youngest went to school she discovered chat rooms where she found it very interesting to talk to different people from all over the world. Before long, she was hooked. What started out as 'innocent' online flirting soon ended up as serial cyber sex. She admitted that she loved the attention she was getting from the men she met online – something she felt was missing in her own marriage. But deep down she didn't like what was happening either. That's when she came for help. Luckily, she decided to end her online liaisons and begin addressing the problems in her marriage that had been festering for some time. So far, her story has a happy ending. Will yours?

What you need to do

Giving up something you enjoy is never easy to do. If you've ever tried to quit smoking or cut down your alcohol use or food intake, you'll know there is no magic cure. Often when people come to see us for help with a certain problem they hope that we'll be able to wave our magic wand and 'cure' them. The harsh reality is that no-one else can do it for you, it's up to you. We know from our work as psychologists that following a program that looks at both your behaviour and your thinking is necessary to make any kind of change in your life.

Change will not happen overnight. To successfully alter your behaviour you have to be prepared to put in the necessary groundwork, develop your action plan, enlist appropriate support and then take small steps. Evaluating your progress and making changes as you go is vital. Also, it's important from the outset to examine your expectations about how easily you'll be able to make changes. We see many people who become disheartened and 'throw in the towel' because they expected to make changes quickly without any tough times. We think it is fair to say that the longer you have been hooked on the Net and the greater dependence you feel on it, the more difficult it will be to make the changes. That, however, is no reason to give up. You just have to expect a few false starts and some rough patches along the way.

Hopefully by now you have some understanding about the warning signs of excessive Internet use. Knowing when to get offline is really important and takes a lot of guts. We're now going to take an in-depth look at our self-help program that we believe can assist those of you who feel your Internet use is out of hand.

In brief ...

- Excessive Internet use is a growing problem.
- If you find it hard to get offline, you could have a problem with your Internet behaviour.
- If you're online for more than three hours each day then you could have a problem.
- Some people who use the Net to excess are avoiding something else in their life.

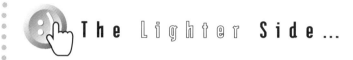

The Lighter Side...

Why TV is better than the Internet

1. It doesn't take minutes to build the picture when you change TV channels.

2. When was the last time you tuned into 'Sea Change' and got a 'Not Found 404' message?

3. There are fewer grating colour schemes on TV – even on MTV.

4. The family never argues over which website to visit this evening.

5. A remote control has fewer buttons than a keyboard.

6. Even the worst TV shows never excuse themselves with an 'Under Construction' sign.

7. 'Seinfeld' never slows down when a lot of people tune in.

8. You just can't find those cool 'Good Morning Australia' exercise-machine infomercials on the Net.

9. Set-top boxes don't beep and whine when you hook up to Foxtel.

10. You can't surf the Net from a couch with a beer in one hand and a pizza slice in the other.

9 The program

We have covered a lot of ground and outlined many strategies to help people change their thinking and behaviour about their Internet use. Now we'll look closely at the steps required to help you break the cycle of excessive Internet use. In this chapter, we'll take you step by step through our self-help program for Internet problems. Keep in mind, however, that we are presenting you with the basics and that you'll need to tailor the program to your own specific set of circumstances. That's why we think following the program in conjunction with treatment from a clinical psychologist is the best approach.

Our self-help program

We have based our program on the psychological techniques we would use if you were to walk through our door requesting help for your Internet use. The core program will take you a minimum of four weeks to complete. After that you will continue working on your own goals, and in that sense you become your own psychologist.

For each week, we list the aims for what we want you to achieve and the tasks you need to complete before you move onto the next week. If you find these tasks take you a little longer, that's okay. In particular we will be focusing on how you behave and what you think. Eventually these levels are tackled at the same time, so it's probably a good idea to read through the whole program first so that you have an idea where we are heading.

As we'll be asking you to complete a number of exercises, we recommend you record your answers in a diary or notebook to keep them together. This way you can easily chart your progress.

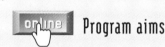 **Program aims**

The overall aims of the self-help program are:

1. to help you identify what triggers your excessive Internet use.

2. to help you learn skills to manage your Internet use.

3. to help you maintain a healthy sense of control in your life.

Week 1: Owning the problem

Aims:

1. to admit you have a problem with your Internet use

2. to acknowledge that you want to do something to change it

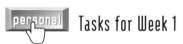 **Tasks for Week 1**

1. Complete the following exercises from this section –
   Whose problem is it? Your Internet path and
   Do I want to change my Internet behaviour? ▶

2. Record all your Internet activity in your Internet diary for the entire week.

3. Read Chapter 8 of *Online and Personal*.

Let's now look more closely at what you are trying to achieve in your first week. If you are at the point of seriously wanting to do something about your problem, you have to be able to admit to yourself first that your Internet behaviour is a problem for you and those closest to you. Without admitting that it is **your** problem, you will always have an out to deflect the responsibility for your behaviour onto something or someone else.

Now, in relation to your Internet activity or activities, complete the following exercise.

personal **Whose problem is it?**

○ Write down which Internet activities are causing you concern?

○ Complete the following statement: *Yes, I admit my Internet behaviour is out of control because it interferes with* _____

_____

_____

It also is useful to understand how you got to where you are. The following questions might help you do this.

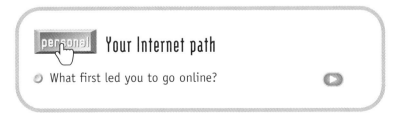

personal **Your Internet path**

○ What first led you to go online?

- What activity did you try first?
- Is that the same activity that you are now having trouble managing? If not, how did you become interested in your problem activity?
- Can you identify when your Internet behaviour started to get out of control? What was happening for you at that time?
- What's your understanding as to why your Internet behaviour is now out of control?

Being clear about why you went online in the first place is important in helping you overcome your excessive Internet use. If it was because you were lonely, for example, that helps you highlight where you will need to focus some of your attention, even if you're not lonely now. It will be important to have thought about what you can do next time you feel lonely instead of logging onto the Internet. Similarly, being aware of when you started to feel out of control about your Internet activity can help you work out what safeguards you need to put in place in case you ever are confronted with similar situations again.

Commitment to change

Even though you might have admitted that your Internet behaviour is a problem, you need to be committed to the process of change in your own mind. Completing the following exercise will help clarify your level of commitment to change. When answering these questions, be specific about which Internet activity you are referring to. For example, your use of pornography, cyber sex, interactive games, general surfing, chat rooms, online gambling or online shopping. If you are involved with more than one activity, begin with the one you believe interferes with your life the most, then the next, and so on.

Do I want to change my Internet behaviour?

Internet activity _____

- What do I enjoy about my Internet use?
- What don't I enjoy about my Internet use?
- What do I gain from my Internet use?
- What does my Internet use prevent me from doing?
- What would I like to keep the same about my Internet use?
- What would I like to change about my Internet use?

Now answer the tricky question about your level of commitment. Be honest with yourself.

On a scale from 0 to 10, choose the number that best represents how committed you are to changing your specific Internet use.

0	1	2	3	4	5	6	7	8	9	10
not committed										totally committed

If you answered 7 or less to the last question we would probably tell you we don't think you are ready to embark on a program to change your behaviour. In our experience, people who score less than 7 or 8 tend to bail out too easily when the going gets tough. If you fall into this category we recommend you read the rest of this book, then answer these questions again. Without a near perfect score of 10, you can try every strategy in this book without any long-term success at cutting back your Internet use.

Observing your behaviour

If you think you are ready to commit yourself to trying the program, it is important to have a clear picture of what exactly it is you are trying to change. For that reason we ask you to do two things. The first is to keep a record of your Internet use for one week, starting now. The second is to list the circumstances or situations that trigger your urge to go online. Below is an example of an Internet diary for you to copy. Your initial entry becomes your 'baseline' measure from which you can chart your progress. If for some reason the week you start recording is not a typical week, we recommend you continue for another week to ensure you have an accurate picture of your use. Start recording your Internet use from Day 1 of Week 1. Whenever you go online fill in all columns except the time you stopped. Do this when you log off, so keep your Internet diary near your computer.

1. Internet diary

Date	Time started	Time stopped	Internet activity	Urge (0–10)
18 Oct	7.00 p.m.	11.30 p.m.	chatting to online friends	7
18 Oct	11.30 p.m.	2.00 a.m.	viewing porn and masturbating	10

Some of you may be surprised to see how much time you actually spend online. People tend to underestimate their Internet use so writing it down is an important step in changing your behaviour pattern. Even though you may feel uncomfortable writing down your activities, you need to be completely honest, otherwise you're not really helping yourself in the long run.

The last column refers to your urge to partake in your online activities. By urge, we mean a persistent desire or want to perform your Internet activity in order to alleviate tension or discomfort of some kind. Use the following scale to help you rate the strength of your urge for each activity where 0 is no urge and 10 is your maximum urge.

This question should be answered regularly throughout the program as it reflects your progress and highlights any potential trouble spots. In the example above you can see that a stronger urge exists by this person to go online to view pornography. In general, not only are we looking for a reduction in hours or a change in Internet behaviour, but a decreased urge to go online.

How strong is my urge?

How strong is my urge to go online and do X? Select the number that best reflects this urge and record it in your diary.

0	1	2	3	4	5	6	7	8	9	10

no
urge

maximum
urge

2. Trigger diary

It is also important to gain a good understanding of what triggers your excessive Internet use. A trigger is anything that sets off the chain of events that leads you to go online. It might be a thought, an emotion, a physical sensation or an image. Following the example below, list the things that trigger your urge to go online. In the last column rate the strength of your urge to perform the activity where 0 is no urge and 10 is your maximum urge.

Example

	Trigger	Urge rating 0–10
1.	being alone at home with nothing to do	8
2.	seeing my computer turned off at home	3
3.	seeing my computer turned on at home	5
4.	feeling sexually aroused	7
5.		
6.		
7.		
8.		
9.		
10.		

Week 2: Changing your behaviour

Aims:

1. to set specific goals for the changes you want to make
2. to begin to implement those changes

 Tasks for Week 2

1. Complete the exercise in this section, **How would you like to act?**
2. Decide whether you want to limit or eliminate your problem Internet behaviour.
3. Identify your goals and define the steps you need to take to achieve these goals by answering **Set your goals**.
4. Choose the competing behaviours for the Internet activity you are targeting from our list **Examples of competing behaviours for Internet use**
5. Begin implementing your program.
6. Continue to record your Internet use in your Internet diary.

Let's now look at how you are going to start changing your online behaviour. You most likely already have some idea of how you'd like to be different. Being clear about what you want to change is really important. Setting goals is the next step. To do this, you need to decide what you would like to change about your Internet behaviour. Then you decide how you are going to change it. For some of you it may be reducing the time you spend online playing games, for others it may be cutting out your use of pornography. Whether you have one goal or several, the key is to keep your goals small and specific.

Setting your goals

Now we want you to think about what you'd like to change. It's important to be clear in your own mind how you would like to be in relation to your Internet behaviour.

How would you like to act?

- What is the Internet activity you would like to change? *e.g. interactive games*
- Describe your average current use of this activity? *Start playing at about 8 p.m. each weeknight and quit about 12 midnight – i.e. 20 hours/week. Don't play on weekend because too busy.*
- Describe how you would like to act in relation to this activity? *Play these games during the week for a maximum of two hours, four times per week – i.e. 8 hours/week.*

You need to be realistic about your goals. Do you want to cut down on your problem Internet activity or eliminate it altogether? Cutting down or controlling your problem Internet behaviour can be difficult because of its accessibility and the fact that you may need to use the Net for work. You might like to try to cut down your behaviour at first then try eliminating it next time. Some behaviours are easier to control than others. General surfing, for example, could be cut down so that you limit your sessions to particular days only. If your Internet problem involves a sexual activity, however, we think abstinence from that activity is the best way to go.

We offer a word of caution, however. In our experience people who do several things online find it hard if they aren't consistent in how they tackle all of their activities. For example, if you want to cut out cyber sex from your Internet life, allowing yourself to frequent X-rated chat rooms is probably setting yourself up to fail. Why? Because there will always be triggers that are likely to start the ball rolling. It might not be today but eventually you could get to the point where you think: *Oh, what the heck!* The general rule is – make your Internet activities as separate as possible. Deciding by location might be one strategy that works for you. For example, use the Internet at work for work-related activities but not at home. In this way, you're changing your environment so that it works for you rather than against you. Before you can take these seemingly drastic steps, the negative impact from your Internet activity needs to outweigh the benefits you gain from doing it.

What's important to remember is that what works for one won't necessarily work for all. Usually, a certain amount of trial and error is needed. One rule of thumb is that if something is really a problem for you, work towards eliminating it from your life. In our experience it's all too easy to regress and before you know it one hour turns into ten, and chatting turns into cyber sex.

A note about sleeping patterns: If your sleep pattern has been disturbed by your Internet use, it's going to take a while to get back to normal; so be prepared for some wakeful nights. Have a novel by your bed, or the hot milk waiting. But whatever you do, don't use it as a reason to get back online. Remember, the key is all in your thinking – eventually your sleep will return to normal if you give it a chance. If sleeplessness is one of your triggers then you need to address this problem too.

Let's now look at some different suggestions depending on whether or not you want to (i) limit your Internet activity or (ii) eliminate it altogether.

Limiting your Internet use

Before you embark on strategies to help you limit your online behaviour, you need to set very specific, well-defined goals. Let's use the earlier example. This person wants to get to the point where he only plays games four times each week for a maximum of two hours each time. It's a big leap, however, to go from twenty hours to eight hours all in one step. So we'd suggest he do something like the following. (His goal-setting starts in Week 2 as in Week 1 he recorded his Internet activity in his Internet diary).

Set your goals

Have a look at this example and then set your own goals.

Target goal: *Play these games for two hours, four times per week, i.e. 8 hours.*

Steps required to achieve this goal:

1. On Day 1 of Week 2, start playing on weeknights at 8 p.m. but finish at 11 p.m. (*5 x 3 = 15 hours*).

2. Introduce one 'games-free' night in the third week, planning a special activity instead (*4 x 3 = 12 hours*).

3. Start playing at 8 p.m. but finish at 10 p.m. in the fourth week (*4 x 2 = 8 hours*), keeping one weeknight 'games free'.

Obviously, you might have to adjust your goals if you find the steps are too small or too big. Most people may need an extra week or two to include more steps to reach their goal; that's perfectly okay. If you manage to achieve the first step, you're going to feel good about that and will be encouraged to keep going. The following guidelines will also help you stick to the limits you have set yourself. But a word of caution, keep your expectations about change realistic. If you've struggled for a long time on your own with your Internet use, it's going to take time and lots of hard work and you'll most likely encounter a few hiccups along the way. If you expect them, you won't be too hard on yourself when they happen. If you slip and find yourself back online, the key is to pick up the ***next day*** exactly where you would have been in your program – don't let yourself think: *Well, I've blown it now, I'll restart the program next week.* It's far better to think: *Slip-ups are a normal part of learning new ways to manage this problem. I can learn from my mistakes. Now, what do I need to plan for tomorrow?*

Guidelines for limiting your Internet use

- List the positives and negatives of your Internet use.
- Work out ahead of time your goals for change.
- Plan your weekly Internet use.
- Schedule other enjoyable activities – see our 'competing behaviours' list
- Include at least two computer-free days per week.
- Set time limits, e.g. two hours maximum per day for recreational use.
- Go online for a specific reason only – avoid surfing from site to site.
- Use an alarm clock to limit your online session time.
- Change your Internet Service Provider plan to one that limits your hours per month.
- Only use your computer at work for work-related activities.
- Keep an accurate diary of your Internet use.
- Use clear thinking to ward off unhelpful thoughts that keep you online.
- Develop an action plan ahead of time if you find yourself in danger of slipping backwards.
- Seek the help of your family or friends.
- If you find you can't limit it alone, seek professional help.

If online shopping is your problem behaviour, you'll have to be creative as to the limits you set. Restricting your credit limit to a very small amount may be one option. Other options might include having only one credit card, or shopping only at one e-store. However, because compulsive online shopping can be so financially damaging, we encourage you to seek professional treatment with someone who is experienced in this type of problem.

Eliminating your Internet use

It is unrealistic to cease all Internet-related activities as the Internet is so much a part of our lives. But we recommend working towards eliminating your problem Internet activity if any areas of your life are at risk, as indicated by any of the warning signs listed below.

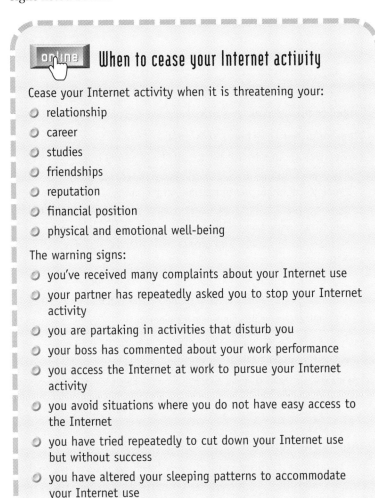

online **When to cease your Internet activity**

Cease your Internet activity when it is threatening your:

○ relationship
○ career
○ studies
○ friendships
○ reputation
○ financial position
○ physical and emotional well-being

The warning signs:

○ you've received many complaints about your Internet use
○ your partner has repeatedly asked you to stop your Internet activity
○ you are partaking in activities that disturb you
○ your boss has commented about your work performance
○ you access the Internet at work to pursue your Internet activity
○ you avoid situations where you do not have easy access to the Internet
○ you have tried repeatedly to cut down your Internet use but without success
○ you have altered your sleeping patterns to accommodate your Internet use
○ you are spending more than you can afford on Internet-related activities

If you decide you want to try and eliminate a certain Internet behaviour then you need to follow the recommendations for limiting Internet use in the previous section. Setting your target goals is your next step. Here is an example to give you some suggestions. Obviously there are many, many combinations and you'll need to work out the best one for you.

 Set your goals

Have a look at this example and then set your own goals.

Target goal: *To completely cut out my use of porn.*

Steps required to achieve this goal:

1. Be clear about why I want to cut it out of my life.
2. From my Internet diary and trigger diary completed in Week 1, highlight my potential trouble spots.
3. Plan for the second week exactly what I'll do in the time I would normally have been online. For example: Monday night – go to movies and dinner with friends; Tuesday night – tennis, etc.
4. Remove all pornographic material from my computer*.
5. Introduce one night at home alone in the third week.
6. Introduce two nights at home in Week 4.
7. Challenge my unhelpful thinking.
8. Attend a support group.

* Be prepared to remove computer from home if too hard to keep out of adult chat rooms and the like.

Change your routine

Before you try to eliminate or limit any behaviour in your life that takes up a significant amount of your time, you need to know what you are going to put in its place. It is best to find something that is difficult to do at the same time as the behaviour you are trying to change. We refer to this as a competing behaviour. We have listed a number for you to give you some ideas. For example, if you want to cut down your time playing online games, you need to ask yourself, what else could I do *in that time* that I enjoy and has nothing to do with either the Internet or a computer?

Exercise is a competing behaviour that many people find easy to do. If you have typically gone online after dinner, changing your routine is crucial. Make sure you are dressed in your exercise gear before eating, then either have a friend collect you or leave the home immediately. Doing something that makes you feel good is really important. Some of you might be saying: *I tried that and it didn't work for very long.* But remember, we are presenting a program that has a number of levels, and it is important to be working on all levels at any one time. Often we find people come unstuck because while they do change their behaviour initially, their thinking is often left unaltered. We teach many of our clients to use the technique of clear thinking that we outline in the next section.

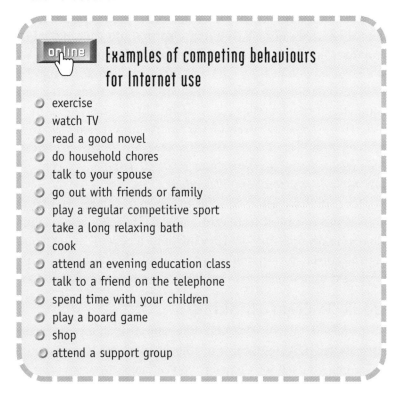

online Examples of competing behaviours for Internet use

- exercise
- watch TV
- read a good novel
- do household chores
- talk to your spouse
- go out with friends or family
- play a regular competitive sport
- take a long relaxing bath
- cook
- attend an evening education class
- talk to a friend on the telephone
- spend time with your children
- play a board game
- shop
- attend a support group

Chart your progress and reward yourself

In the second week, continue to record your Internet use in your diary even though you will be attempting to change your behaviour now according to the goals you have set yourself. Clearly mark when your intervention actually started, keep a record of what your target goals were and the competing behaviours you substituted. This is particularly useful so you can see your progress. It also helps identify the weak spots in your program and where you may need to make some changes. Even if you don't go online, record the activity you wanted to do and how strong your urge was to go online in the last column. Put an asterisk next to it to indicate that you didn't go online. Write down what you did instead. It's really important at that point to *resist the urge* to go online. If you can let that desire wash over you, you'll most likely find the urge will lessen. Try and get on with your normal activities and give the urge a chance to subside.

When you first try to make changes you may feel irritable and depressed; that's normal. You may also slip into your old habits and that's normal too. If ever you feel you're slipping, try to delay when you go online. Even if it's only for fifteen minutes, it may be enough time for the urge to subside. Do something from our competing behaviours list. Call a friend, have a bath or go for a run. These activities give you an opportunity to change your thinking from: *I need to go online. I can't do this, it's all too hard*, to *I can choose not to go online. Instead I'll call X and have a chat. If I take this one step at a time, I'll get there.*

Once you have achieved some of the goals you set, no matter how small, you need to reward yourself. Decide ahead of time what your rewards may be. They might be a new CD, a night out, or a long distance telephone call to a friend. They don't have to be large, just something that helps you acknowledge your progress.

Week 3: Clear thinking

By the beginning of Week 3, you should be clear about your goals, have started making changes to your Internet behaviour, and be rewarding yourself for the gains you've made. Now we want to spend some time on your thinking. Even if you're doing really well so far, the skill of clear thinking is helpful when you start to find the going a bit tough.

Aims:
1. to begin a diary of your thoughts
2. to learn how to challenge your unhelpful thinking

 Tasks for Week 3

1. Record in your diary your A-B-Cs as outlined in this section.
2. After the fact, attempt to complete the Ds and Es in your diary.
3. Continue to record your Internet behaviour in your Internet diary.
4. Continue to follow your goals, using competing behaviours.

If you are dependent on the Internet, you need to look closely at your thinking patterns. Clear thinking is a skill we teach a lot of people who walk through our door, regardless of their problem. It is based on the premise that *the way you think influences the way you feel and how you behave*. The clear thinking component of the program is crucial to your progress as it provides an opportunity to choose a different way of behaving.

What is clear thinking?

Before we look at what you need to do yourself, let's look at the following example: Jenny, Kate and Stephen are at a lunch. Their host tells them that a mutual friend has recently left her husband and children for a man she met on the Internet. This news makes Jenny feel sad, Kate indifferent and Stephen angry. The news of the separation does not in fact *cause* the feelings in each of these people, but rather triggers different thoughts that cause different feelings.

Jenny feels sad because she *thinks* of her unhappy childhood after her parents divorced. Kate is unaffected by the news because she *thinks* about how happy she is since her recent marriage. Stephen is angry because he *thinks* their friend is selfish and is doing irreparable damage to her children. *It's clear that the different ways these people thought about their friend's separation caused different emotions in each of them.*

Consider another example. Jane and Karen are Internet friends. Jane lives in America and Karen in Australia. They have developed a very close friendship and communicate daily on the Net. Karen, however, occasionally feels a little jealous when Jane tells her about some of her other conversations on the Net when she is asleep in Australia. One particular day Jane does not log on at their usual time. Karen immediately feels angry and jealous. She thinks Jane has forgotten about her and is off chatting to one of her new American Internet pals. When she finally does hear from Jane, Jane tells her that she had spent the night in hospital with her daughter who had hurt herself playing sport at school. What happens to Karen's anger and jealousy? It disappears and Karen almost instantly feels guilty and disappointed in herself for doubting Jane's friendship.

Automatic thinking

Thinking is a very automatic process. You won't always be conscious of your exact thoughts. It's a bit like driving a car; you are not always aware of how you got from one place to the next. So in order to change your feelings and behaviour, you first of all need to identify your thoughts. We encourage people to get into the habit of exploring the reasons why they feel any negative emotion. The reason will usually be some kind of negative or unhelpful thought pattern. In the case of excessive Internet use, we believe that some of you may have gone online initially for work or out of curiosity but soon began to rely on the Internet to soothe yourself. Maybe you feel sad, lonely or anxious. However, unless you get into the habit of identifying your thoughts the negative ones will go unchecked. The consequences then can be very damaging not only for yourself but for your loved ones too.

Inaccurate assumptions

Much of your thinking reflects the fact that you each perceive the world in a different way according to the assumptions you make. Your assumptions tend to be the result of your experience. If your partner has recently left you, you are more likely to notice couples in your everyday life. You might also assume that 'all men are bastards' or 'women can't be trusted'.

But danger comes when the assumptions you make are inaccurate. If you base your judgements and ability to solve problems on inaccurate assumptions, you are setting yourself up to fail. In order to improve the way you feel about something in your life, you must identify inaccurate assumptions and then change them.

What causes feelings?

Understanding how your thinking influences your feelings and the way you react is an important step towards taking responsibility for making changes in your own life. Often people mistakenly think and talk as though situations cause the way they feel and behave. Let's look at Karen's situation with Jane from the last section.

*Jane **made** me so angry when she didn't go online when she said she would.*

It is important to understand that no-one can make you feel angry, or any other emotion for that matter. Situations or events trigger the thoughts, assumptions and beliefs that cause you to feel a certain way. Therefore, you need to identify the thoughts that cause the negative emotions or feelings in the first place. In Karen's example she thought:

When Jane didn't go online, I thought she had forgotten me because she has new Internet friends. Then I got angry.

Learning to identify the thoughts that cause the feelings is central to the process of clear thinking.

How to think clearly

We can illustrate how your thoughts affect your feelings and behaviour as follows:

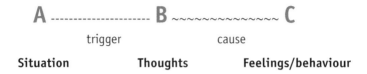

Situation	Thoughts	Feelings/behaviour

In order to change C (your feelings and behaviour), you must change B (your thoughts), and not always look to A (the situation) as the cause of feeling bad. There won't always be an obvious behaviour that follows the thoughts. Sometimes it might just be 'carry on as usual'.

A --------------------- B ~~~~~~~~~~~~~~ C

trigger   cause

Situation	Thoughts	Feelings/behaviour
No message from e-friend	*Where is she? She should be on by now. Maybe she is no longer interested.*	Upset, worried/Teary
No message from e-friend	*She must have got sidetracked. She'll come online soon.*	Neutral/Get on with normal activities

In this example you can see there are at least two ways of thinking about the situation. In fact there are many more ways to think about any given situation. You will feel differently depending on how you ***think*** about the situation. Remember, the situation does not cause the way you feel but rather triggers the thoughts that cause the way you feel.

In order to change the way you feel and what you do, you need to change the way you think. You do this by challenging any unhelpful thoughts once you are aware of them and then changing them into more realistic or helpful thoughts.

We want to show you how unhelpful or negative thoughts can be shifted, even if only slightly. You will probably find you are doing this some of the time. The aim is to become skilled at challenging your unhelpful thoughts most of the time so that you feel more in control of your life and the decisions you make. The desired outcome is to reduce or cut out the Internet behaviour that you believe is affecting your life.

Challenging unhelpful thoughts

We can expand the process in the following way:

A -------- B --------- C --------- D --------- E

| Situation | Thoughts | Feelings/ behaviour | New thoughts | New feelings/ behaviour |

By challenging your thoughts (B), and turning them into new thoughts (D), the aim is to change your feelings and behaviour (E). When people come for therapy about their excessive Internet use they want to change their Cs.

It is important to note that the new thoughts (D) should not be falsely positive, which we would call wishful thinking. They are just realistic. The idea is not to aim for euphoria as a new feeling (E), but rather calmness, or less frustration, or less anxiety. This shift in emotion might then be enough to produce a more helpful and productive behaviour that for some of you will include more reasonable Internet use. For others, it may mean no Internet use at all.

Let's look at an example where a man is having cyber sex with people on the Net because he and his wife are experiencing difficulties in their marriage. He came for help because he was ashamed of what he was doing on the Internet and feared his marriage would end.

A ----------- B ~~~~~~~ C ----------- D ~~~~~~~ E

Situation	Thoughts	Feelings/ behaviour	New thoughts	New feelings/ behaviour
Another argument with wife	*She doesn't give a damn about me or us.*	Angry, sad/ Use chat rooms to meet women online and have cyber sex.	*I don't know what she thinks. Acting this way will make our situation worse. I need to sit down and let her know how I'm feeling so that we can work out something together.*	Less angry, less sad/Set time with wife to talk about problems.

In order to work out the new thoughts, it is often useful to ask yourself the following questions to help you find the realistic thinking that is needed to change the bad feelings or to reduce their intensity. The aim is to ensure that your new thinking is realistic, helpful and flexible. Clear thinking helps you to solve your difficult issues, and in turn is more likely to generate constructive behaviour.

- Where's the evidence for what I thought in B?
- What are the alternatives to what I thought in B?
- What is the likely effect on me of thinking this way?
- How would I advise a friend to think in the same situation?
- How would someone advise me?

When you begin challenging your unhelpful thoughts in this way, select simple situations not major events. Choose an occasion when you felt a negative emotion. It doesn't have to be related to your Internet behaviour at first. In fact it is probably easier to start off with some small, less complicated examples. Perhaps you were running late for work, having a disagreement or doing an errand. Remember, the situation is just the trigger not the cause of your negative emotion. Then, after you have had a few attempts, think back to the last time you went online when you did not want to. What was happening for you? Try to remember what you were thinking at the time.

 Challenge your thoughts

1. Think of a recent situation after which you went online. For example: *Had a bad day at work and came home and went online viewing porn and masturbating.*

2. Use the A-B-C-D-E model to identify your unhelpful thoughts, feelings and behaviour. Try to come up with the new, helpful thoughts in an attempt to change your feelings and particularly your behaviour.

A --------- **B** ~~~~~~ **C** ----------- **D** ~~~~~~~ **E**

Situation	Thoughts	Feelings/ behaviour	New thoughts	New feelings/ behaviour
Bad day at work.	*Who cares? This is all to difficult.*	Annoyed, flat/Go online to view porn	*It doesn't help me to take my work problems home. Tomorrow I'll go and see my boss to talk about it.*	Less annoyed/ Write down what I want to say to boss. Call a friend.

Challenging your thinking is a skill that should be practised daily when you are trying to alter your excessive Internet use. Use it in conjunction with the other skills we have outlined in this chapter. We recommend that you complete the A-B-C-D-E diary format daily for the first three to four weeks. Each time you go online make an entry. Initially, it's easier to practise the exercise after the event; many people tell us it is very hard to identify the negative thoughts, let alone challenge them, when they are feeling awful. If you are having trouble working out what you were thinking in a particular situation, it may help to ask:

- What did I think about myself?
- What did I think about the other people?
- What did I think about the situation itself?

By analysing the sequence of situation-thoughts-feelings/behaviour after the heat of the moment, you can learn from your mistakes. You can then start training your mind to think more realistically and accurately. Like most things, the more you practise challenging your thoughts the easier it will be. Once you get the hang of what you are doing, you can ease up on writing down all the examples in which your negative emotion or reaction was particularly intense. In time the challenging will become more automatic and you will notice your thinking is more helpful, most of the time.

Being able to identify and change the unhelpful thoughts that lead you to go online when you don't want to is a vital component of your program. You will probably have a few lapses as you go but as we said before, make a diary entry so you can examine where you came unstuck. Even though it might seem tedious to complete this exercise on a regular basis, we believe it is a valuable skill to learn. At first, keeping a diary might seem awkward but the more effort you put into keeping the diary, the more benefit you will gain. Many people fall into the trap of just doing it in their heads. In our experience, people make more gains if they write down their examples because more cognitive processing is required to put pen to paper.

Let's look at Rick's diary. He sought help for his desire to view porn and to have online sex, which included having cyber sex with numerous people. One of his target goals was to completely cut out having cyber sex as he was beginning a new relationship and was concerned that it would affect his relationship. He also wanted to stop viewing porngraphy. One of his diary entries is set out below:

A---------- B~~~~~~~ C---------- D~~~~~~~ E

Situation	Thoughts	Feelings/behaviour	New thoughts	New feelings/behaviour
Girlfriend out with firends	*What if she meets someone else?*	Worried, upset/ Go online.	*It's good for us to pursue our own interests. There's no evidence she'll leave – she really loves me.*	Less worried and upset/ Visit a friend.

You can see that if Rick had been able to think helpfully (as he did in D) when his girlfriend went out without him, there would have been less chance of him going online only to regret it the next day.

Week 4: Refining your program

Aims:

1. to refine any difficulties in your program
2. to continue working on your goals
3. to build other interests in your life
4. to develop an action plan for trouble spots

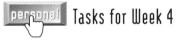 Tasks for Week 4

1. Continue to record your Internet behaviour in your Internet diary.
2. Continue to follow your goals, using competing behaviours.

3. Use clear thinking to challenge your unhelpful thinking – keep your A-B-C-D-E diary.

4. Refine your goals if something isn't working.

5. Prepare your safeguards for any potential trouble spots by completing the **Action plan for trouble exercise** in this section.

6. Set goals for the next month.

7. Complete the **Yearly goals exercise** in this section.

8. Reward yourself for the gains you have made.

Refining your program

If you have followed the program and are having difficulty, you need to go back to your goals and ask yourself:

- Are my goals realistic?
- Am I being too ambitious in what I am trying to achieve?
- Am I setting myself up to fail?
- Do I need to make my steps smaller?
- Am I challenging my unhelpful thinking?

Don't fall into the trap of thinking that all you need is willpower. Making your environment work for you is what counts. We like to explain it this way. A very obese client came for help. She would say: *I just don't have enough willpower – that's my problem.* When asked why she thought that, she replied: *I just can't stop eating ice cream – I love it.* Being reasonable clinicians, we suggested that eating a small serving of ice cream on occasion was okay. But she was buying up big when she saw the large containers of ice cream on sale at the supermarket. When she hit a rough patch she'd eat and eat and eat. It took her a while to realise that managing her weight was far more important to her than the few extra cents she saved by buying the ice cream on sale. Forget the willpower!

We certainly won't pretend that trying to change an established problem behaviour is easy. Use our self-help program as a guide and remember that you'll need to make changes and learn by trial and error. Our four-week core program is only the beginning of the rest of your life. Excessive Internet use is not something that's going to go away for you just because you did what we said for four weeks. You need to see these changes as lifestyle changes. We also can't emphasise enough that if you are taking something out of your life that previously took up a large chunk of time and energy, you need to replace it with something constructive.

Yearly goals

We believe it is really important for anyone's self-esteem to do things that make them feel good. Setting personal goals and working towards achieving them is one way to do this. We suggest you work through the exercise below. If you're in a relationship, you can also complete these goals as a couple as well as individually.

 Yearly goals exercise

1. What would you like to achieve in the next twelve months? Be specific, and consider the following areas:

    - friendships
    - leisure activities
    - fitness
    - career/education
    - finances
    - family (extended)
    - children (if applicable)
    - other

2. What steps do you need to take to achieve the goals you have made?

3. Which goal do you want to target first, second and so on?

Potential trouble spots

When anyone is making huge changes in their lives, they need to be prepared for the times when things aren't going smoothly for them. Probably the most difficult times to keep your Internet use in check will be when you're feeling down, anxious or angry for some reason. But if you're prepared you can plan what you need to do to ward off trouble. Maybe you've got a friend you can call or a telephone counsellor. If there is a support group for Internet users in your local area then you may find that helpful too. Support groups can be a great benefit especially in conjunction with counselling. If there isn't one, maybe you can think about starting up your own. If you're feeling down, we'd recommend that at all costs you keep away from your computer. Don't put yourself in the line of temptation – it's not worth the risk. Remember, the urge to go online will eventually subside if you give it time.

Confronting your triggers

At the end of Week 1 we asked you to list the triggers to your excessive Internet use. Now we want you to go back and look at them again. If you are pleased with the progress you have made so far, it's a good exercise to now face the situations that trigger your desire to go online. This is called *exposure*. Remember we said that not only was a reduction in your Internet behaviour your goal, but also a lessening of your urge to go online. The aim of this exercise is to expose yourself to the urge to use the Net but prevent yourself from going online. In time, the urge will lessen. The graph below outlines what happens to your urge.

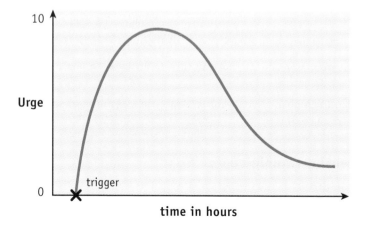

Beginning with the trigger that has the lowest urge rating, set up a situation that allows you to confront that trigger. If we use the example from Week 1, you would tackle *seeing my computer turned off at home (urge score 3)* first. Prepare exactly what you will do in advance so you will be able to challenge your unhelpful thinking and in a way 'psyche' yourself up to confront the task. For example, you could sit in front of the computer and deliberately look at it, and record your urge score at say ten-minute intervals. We would expect your score to go up but then start to lessen in time. It may take you an hour or so to see a significant reduction in the score, but whatever you do, don't turn your computer on. You stay with the task until you notice at least a 50 percent reduction in your urge. Then tackle the next highest *seeing my computer on at home (urge score 5)* and so on. You will have different thoughts going through your head while you're attempting this exercise, which is perfectly normal. Try to remain focused on your thoughts about your Internet use. Distracting yourself with other thoughts is not really facing your triggers. You are also likely to experience discomfort or distress as you face these triggers without allowing yourself to go online. Once again this is normal, and we would expect your level of discomfort to also decrease with time, after an initial peak. Continuing to expose yourself to different triggers is something you could keep doing over the next few weeks.

Your action plan

In preparation for those inevitable tough times complete the following exercise:

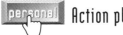 **Action plan for trouble**

1. What are your potential trouble spots?
2. What action do you need to take if you are heading for trouble?

Once you have completed the core program, you'll have the tools necessary to plan your own program for the next month using what we've set out here as a guide. If you hit a rough patch, review this chapter and try to identify where you went wrong and what you need to do differently. Keep evaluating and tailoring your program as you go.

Conclusion

We've armed you with a number of skills that you need to practise regularly and incorporate into your daily routine. You have learnt how to set goals and alter your behaviour by changing what you do, and when you do it. We have outlined the importance of challenging unhelpful thoughts and replacing them with realistic ones, and rewarding yourself for the gains you make along the way. At the end of the day, changing your Internet behaviour won't be easy. But the more you put into it, the more you'll get out of it.

In brief...

- To help yourself you need to admit that your Internet use is a problem.
- Set your goals for what you want to change.
- Develop your action plan.
- Challenge any unhelpful thinking.
- Build new interests.
- There's no magic cure, just hard work.

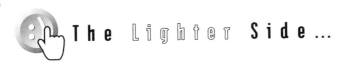

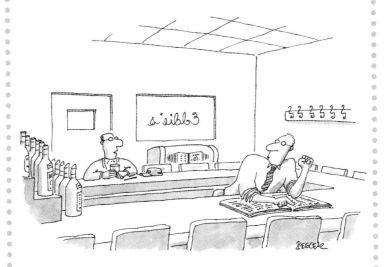

*"To avoid the tedium of this endless socialising, Eddie,
I have decided, beginning Monday, to obtain all my future
booze from Amazon.com."*

10

Moving forward with the Internet

Hopefully by now you have a good idea of what you need to do about the Internet concerns you ticked in Chapter 1. It's up to each of us to manage how the Internet influences our lives both as individuals and as a global society. Moving forward *with* the Internet as opposed to *ignoring* it is the key to success. We are now starting to see the effects of the changes the Internet has brought into our lives – these are widespread; both good and bad. Rather than shying away from these changes we encourage you to work out what you need to do to deal with the impact the Internet is having on your life.

It seems we are all struggling with information overload and the full impact of the Internet in business and relationships is yet to be realised. To move forward, we need a framework to guide our behaviour regarding the Internet. This framework needs to include guidelines for how we think and behave online as individuals and as a society. Naturally, change is going to take time; but it is not time itself that will produce the outcome you want, it is what you do in the time.

Let's finish with our five conclusions

In Chapter 1 we listed the five conclusions we drew from our discussions with people about the Internet. These were:

1. The Internet itself is not the problem – it's how some people use it.
2. Take your time approaching anyone or anything online.
3. Know when to get offline.
4. Internet affairs are affairs.
5. Get informed and take action.

Let's take another look at them now.

Develop your personal code of conduct

When you think about the Internet, it's important to remember that it is simply another communication tool and not some technological monster out to destroy us. The problems we are currently facing as a result of the explosion of the Internet into our lives are not new. It's just that the Internet presents them in a new light and in far greater numbers. People, for example, have always had affairs, accessed inappropriate information or preyed on unsuspecting children, just as teenagers have tested the limits or become consumed by the latest fad. So, where do we go from here?

We are now experiencing a period of transition while the guidelines for acceptable Internet use are defined and modified. We've talked a lot about appropriate behaviour on the Internet for different groups, including adults both single and in relationships, teenagers and children, in our society. It is up to all of us to take on the responsibility of developing a personal code of conduct for appropriate online behaviour, in our working and our private lives, that reflects our society's values. If, for example, you are an employer, you need to define your acceptable Internet use policy and ensure the standards are met. If you're in a relationship then you need to be clear what behaviour reflects your commitment to your partner and what behaviour does not. Similarly, if you're a parent your responsibility is to educate your children about how to behave online. Don't expect your child's school to take on the full responsibility of educating them about the Internet. Your child is online both in and out of school hours and you need to be involved. If you or your children are concerned about something you see on the Internet, act. Inform the appropriate people, be they a chat room host, another parent, the school or the police. Litigation is rapidly catching up to the technology. Parents are beginning to sue site hosts who allow damaging messages to be posted or harassment to go unchecked. As the litigation continues and picks up momentum, the moral and legal codes will be written and rewritten. Until then, constant feedback is needed – both positive and negative.

Whoever you are, it's important to remember that the Internet is a part of real life and we need to play by 'real life' rules. That is, if a behaviour is inappropriate, offensive, or destructive in everyday life then it is inappropriate, offensive or destructive online. There will always be cultural differences. We have to manage these as best as we can within our own society. If you are unsure about the suitability of certain behaviours while you, your children or your partner are on the Net, stop, think and ask yourself: *If this interaction happened with someone face to face, how would I react?*

Even though etiquette exists on the Internet (known as 'netiquette') and includes guidelines for how to behave on the Net, many people are not familiar with these guidelines. We believe we have to take it further and answer some of the tougher questions. People need to start talking and keep talking about how the Internet is affecting their lives. Where, for example, does the free expression of ideas cross the boundary of being discriminatory and offensive to others? Should we regulate or legislate against inaccurate or dangerous information? How do we manage cultural differences? The list is never ending so at the end of the day, it's up to all of us.

Make the Internet part of your life, not all of it

Regardless of what you actually do on the Internet, it's important to ensure that it is only a part of your life, not your entire life. The old saying: 'everything in moderation' is relevant here. If you follow this advice you are less likely to end up in trouble. If you're single and using the Internet as a dating service, be on the lookout for real-life opportunities to meet people as well. If you use the Internet as a way of socialising then the same advice applies. If you've met someone online, bring that relationship into the real world so you can incorporate it into your life as soon as possible. If you can't wait to log on each night after work or school, you probably need to put the brakes on. Don't let it dominate your life or dictate your movements. If you find you're changing your schedule to accommodate your Internet use, we'd say you most likely have some kind of problem and you need to address it now.

Maybe you and the Internet don't mix

From all accounts, there are going to be many people who have a problem with how they use the Internet. If you believe that some aspect of your online behaviour causes you more harm than good, you need to work out how you will structure your environment to keep your behaviour in check. If you think you're hooked on some aspect of the Internet, you need to make a choice – to either limit your usage or eliminate it altogether. Seeking help is your next step, and our self-help program is a good start.

Keep out of the way of temptation

If you're in a committed relationship don't kid yourself that online relationships are okay because 'real' sex hasn't occurred. Internet affairs are not okay. You need to remind yourself about what is appropriate offline behaviour. Where would disclosing personal and intimate details of your life within an intimate context to another person of your partner's sex be permissible? If you find you are 'talking' to someone in particular on the Internet on a regular basis and thinking about them a lot then get offline. It all comes back to accepting responsibility for your own behaviour. The biggest mistake people make about the Internet is failing to see what happens online within the context of 'real' living. You can't separate your online life from your real world life – the same rules of commitment, honesty and trust apply to your relationship, even if you have never met your online partner. If you are talking to someone intimately on the Net, you are not committed to your real-life relationship. If you would not like your partner to be intimate with someone else on or offline, reconsider your behaviour. If you find yourself turning to someone you have met on the Internet, you may need to turn your attention to your relationship and do everything to remain committed to your partner.

Strive to maximise the positives and minimise the negatives

The motto that best sums up our ideas from writing *Online and Personal* has to be **get informed and take action**. No matter what your involvement is with the Internet, this motto is crucial. You might be in business, in a relationship or worried about your children online, but the reality is you can't help if you don't know.

As we've said all along, the Internet itself is not a problem, just how some people use it. To move forward, you need to know how you can maximise the positives and minimise the negatives in relation to the Internet. It's a great way to interact with people, access information and do business. But it's hard to do these things if you don't have a basic understanding of what it all means. It's a bit like driving a car; most of us drive a car without a complete understanding of the intricacies of a motor but we hopefully have some sense of what to do and what not to do. The same applies to the Internet; you don't need to understand the complexities of how it works, just have a sense of the dangers and what you need to do to avoid problems. If you're holding back, a little afraid of the technology, challenge your thoughts that keep you stuck. Work out what you need to do to get informed and take action now. If you're an employer, define appropriate Internet conduct for your staff and ensure that help is available for employees who may have a problem with their Internet use. If you're in a relationship then be open with each other about the 'rules' of your Internet behaviour. If something is irritating you, speak up; your partner can't mind read. If you're a parent, your child no doubt knows more than you do about the Internet; the best thing you can do for them is to keep the communication channels open and teach them to act in a way that reflects your family's and society's values.

The Internet is the future. The best advice we can offer is to remember that the Internet is a fabulous communication tool, but at the end of the day, how you use the Internet is up to you.

Authors' notes

Page ix **Cognitive Behaviour Therapy** – For a comprehensive discussion see either:

> Beck, A.T., *Cognitive Therapy and the Emotional Disorders* International Universities Press, New York, 1976.
>
> or
>
> Ellis, A. and Harper, R.A., *A New Guide to Rational Living.* Wilshire Book Company, Hollywood, 1975.

Chapter One: The Internet – the good, the bad and the ugly

Page 2 **computer network connecting millions of computers...** – This definition is taken from Booth, A., *Making the Internet Work for your Business,* Allen and Unwin, Sydney, 1999.

Page 2 **psychologists are struggling to keep up with the development of the Internet.** – Psychological research into Internet addiction and how the Internet is affecting people's lives is in its infancy. Psychological and psychiatric circles are divided as to whether or not Internet addiction is a new, discrete psychological disorder. For more information see Holliday, H. 'Hooked on the net', *Psychology Today,* (2000), vol. 33, p. 10; and Mitchell, P., 'Internet addiction: genuine diagnosis or not?', *The Lancet,* (2000), vol. 355, p. 632.

Page 9 **technological generation gap** – We coined this term to describe the pattern that is emerging where children know more than their parents about certain technologies. These technologies include computers in general, TV and video equipment, electronic games and the Internet. As a result of this technological generation gap, traditional roles are reversed between parents and children because parents in many cases are reliant on their children to use the technology. In turn, parents start losing control over their children's behaviour because of their limited knowledge, and the children are more likely to outsmart them about what they are doing. The term is also relevant to other areas, such as designer drugs, where the gap between parents' and children's knowledge is increasing.

Page 9 **six percent of Internet users are addicted** – This estimate was reported in Greenfield, D., *Virtual Addiction: help for netheads, cyberfreaks, and those who love them*, New Harbinger, Oakland, 1999. Dr Greenfield's book provides a detailed look at the nature of compulsive Internet use. From his research into Internet use, Dr Greenfield estimates that six percent of Internet users are addicted. Dr Greenfield (see p. 66) distinguishes between abuse and addiction, and has developed the Internet Abuse Test and Virtual Addiction Test. He says that the main difference is that an abuser doesn't appear to suffer from tolerance or withdrawal, and tends not to experience as many serious consequences of their behaviour as an addict does. Abusers can learn to change the way they use the Internet.

Page 9 **excessive Internet use** – We prefer to use the descriptive term 'excessive Internet use' rather than Internet addiction in *Online and Personal*, given that no formal psychiatric diagnosis currently exists for Internet addiction. We are particularly concerned with anyone whose life in some way is being adversely affected by their Internet use.

Page 10 **acceptable use** – Acceptable use policies or guidelines are terms used to describe acceptable Internet behaviour. These terms are particularly relevant in schools, and refer to the guidelines and standards for how the Internet is to be used.

Page 11 **The Ugly Side** – See Aftab, P., *The Parent's Guide to Protecting your Children in Cyberspace*, McGraw-Hill, New York, 2000. This book is an excellent source of information about children and teenagers on the Net, especially covering topics such as hate sites, paedophiles and harassment.

Page 11 **Cyber crime is on the increase** – This statement was made in an article by Kong, D. and Swartz, J., 'Experts see rash of heart attacks coming' in *USA Today*, 27/9/00.

Chapter Two: The difference between conventional and Internet relationships

Page 20 **bubble stage** – For a more in-depth discussion, see Lamble, J. and Morris, S., *Side by Side: How to think differently about your relationship*, Finch Publishing, Sydney, 2000.

Page 22 **commitment** – See our previous book, ibid., for a more detailed explanation of commitment and why it is the first step towards a successful relationship.

Chapter Three: Singles on the Net

Page 31 **Internet dating services are on the increase** – This statement was taken from an article by Stephanie Stroughton, 'Log on, Find love' in the *Boston Sunday Globe,* 11/2/01.

Page 43 **Single person's 'don't' list** – This list has been compiled from our work with clients, discussions with people who have met online, and advice found in Greenfield, op. cit., Aftab, op. cit., and Young, K.S., *Caught in the net: how to recognize the signs of Internet addiction – and a winning strategy for recovery,* John Wiley & Sons, New York, 1998.

Chapter Four: Is the Internet affecting your relationship?

Page 62 **Warning signs that your partner may be involved with someone on the Internet** – We have developed this list, which is by no means exhaustive, from our work with clients and our discussions with people who have met someone online while in a committed relationship, and from advice found in Greenfield, op. cit., and Young, op. cit.

Page 69 **compulsive online gambling and shopping** – See Greenfield, op. cit. for more information about shopping and investing online and the associated problems.

Chapter Five: Help for committed relationships

Page 79 **Clear thinking** – We provide a detailed discussion of clear thinking and how to apply it to your relationships in Lamble and Morris, op. cit. Clear thinking is our user-friendly term to describe cognitive behaviour therapy.

Page 87 **OCEAN Model** – See our previous book, ibid., for more information.

Chapter Six: Teenagers on the Net

Page 94 **Teenagers on the Net** – For a comprehensive review of the problems and dangers facing children on the Internet, and a list of useful website addresses, see Aftab, op. cit., or visit her website, www.familyguidebook.com

Page 103 **A recent conference on prejudice on the Internet** – This conference was reported in an article by Catherine Keenan, 'Hate weaves its web on the Internet' in the *Sydney Morning Herald*, 6/11/00.

Page 104 **Global peer pressure** – We coined this term to refer to a new form of peer pressure where children and teens via the Internet may be influenced by children from all over the world.

Page 107 **Technological generation gap** – See note to Chapter One.

Chapter Seven: Advice for parents

Page 116 **Ways to get informed** was compiled from our work with clients and advice given in Aftab, op. cit. and Young, op. cit.

Page 117 **Ways to take action** was compiled from our work with clients and advice given in Aftab, op cit. and Young, op. cit.

Page 118 **Katie.com –** A must-read for parents and teenagers alike about the dangers of children meeting people on the Internet. See Tarbox, K., *Katie.com,* Dutton, New York, 2000.

Page 123 **Some ground rules** – These are just a few; others can be found in Aftab, op. cit., Tarbox, ibid., and Young, op. cit.

Page 129 **Danger signs of teenager addiction** – These signs are taken from Young, ibid., who offers suggestions to help teenagers who may be addicted to the Internet.

Page 130 **1.5 hours of surfing** – This specific guideline was taken from Parry Aftab's 'teenangels' group. More details can be found in her book Aftab, op. cit.

Page 130 **'Screen' time** – More ideas about limiting screen time, covering television, computers and the Internet, can be found in Dr Christopher Green's recent book *Beyond Toddlerdom – keeping five- to twelve-year-olds on the rails,* Doubleday, Sydney, 2000.

Page 131 **General advice to parents** – We have developed this list from our work with clients and from advice found in Aftab, op. cit. and Young, op. cit.

Chapter Eight: Are you hooked?

Page 137 **Warning signs** – We have developed this general list from our work with clients. This list is not a diagnostic tool. While no formal diagnostic criteria – as defined in the *Diagnostic and statistical manual of mental disorders, 4th edition*, American Psychiatric

Association, Washington DC, 1994 – exist for Internet addiction, some researchers have developed self-report questionnaires to assess a person's dependency on the Internet. For more information, see the Internet Abuse Test (IAT) and the Virtual Addiction Test (VAT) by Greenfield, op. cit., at www.virtual-addiction.com; and the Internet Addiction Test by Young, op. cit., at www.netaddiction.com

Page 141 **What are people avoiding? Top-ten list of avoidances** – This list is taken from Young, op. cit.

Chapter Nine: The program

Page 145 **The program** – Our self-help program draws on a number of cognitive and behavioural techniques that we know work with other types of problems, including eating disorders, compulsive gambling, drug and alcohol problems and the anxiety disorders. We are currently using this approach with clients who come to see us for excessive Internet use, and are aware that the program has yet to be experimentally validated. Given that research into this problem is still in its infancy, we would welcome any comments to help us continue to refine our program. You can contact us at LambleMorris@bigpond.com.

Page 160 **Clear thinking** – This approach is based on the psychological model known as Cognitive Behaviour Therapy (CBT). For a more detailed discussion of CBT see Ellis and Harper, op. cit.

Page 166 **Questions used to challenge your unhelpful thinking** – These questions are based on discussions found in Greenberger, D. and Padesky, C., *Mind Over Mood – change how you feel by changing the way you think*, Guildford Press, New York, 1995; and Andrews, G., Crino, R., Hunt, C., Lampe, L. and Page, A., *The Treatment of Anxiety Disorders*, Cambridge University Press, Melbourne, 1994.

Page 172 **Confronting your triggers** – Clinicians could expand this exercise to cover a more detailed explanation of exposure and response prevention. Subjective units of discomfort scale (SUDS) scores could be introduced and the different components – cognitive, emotional and physical – of a client's urge score defined.

Chapter Ten: Moving forward with the Internet

Page 178 **netiquette** – Many books talk about netiquette; see Aftab, op. cit. for recent guidelines.

Acknowledgements

We would like to thank the many people in both Australia and the United States who answered our questions, told us their stories and shared their experiences and concerns about the Internet. Their contribution makes *Online and Personal* unique and about real people 'out there'.

We are also grateful to Kathryn Kirkwood for her comments and suggestions about the program.

Rex Finch once again gave us a wonderful opportunity, and he and Sean Doyle led us through the many phases of producing this book. A very big thank you also to Marie-Louise Taylor, Sonia Woo and Di Murray, Julianne Sheedy and Debbie McInnes, who were all involved in the editing, design and marketing of *Online and Personal*.

We would also like to thank our family and friends – especially Andrew and David – for their encouragement and support.

We can be contacted at lamblemorris@bigpond.com

Jo Lamble and Sue Morris

<188>

What is a clinical psychologist?

Clinical psychologists help people identify and change unhelpful behaviours and thinking patterns. They use a variety of techniques including interviews, observation and tests. There are many treatment approaches and techniques from which a clinical psychologist will select, according to the presenting problem.

Clinical psychologists are specialist psychologists with a minimum of six years' full-time university training. All practising psychologists must be registered with their State or Territory Registration Board.

Clinical psychologists help prevent, assess, diagnose and treat a wide range of problems encountered by children, adolescents and adults. Common areas of treatment include alcohol and drug problems, anxiety disorders, behavioural difficulties, chronic pain, depression, eating disorders, grief, relationship difficulties, trauma reactions and stress.

For more information about where to find a clinical psychologist, contact the Australian Psychological Society or the New Zealand College of Clinical Psychologists.

Further reading

Aftab, P., *The Parent's Guide to Protecting your Children in Cyberspace*, McGraw-Hill, New York, 2000.

American Psychiatric Association, *Diagnostic and Statistical Manual of Mental Disorders*, 4th edition, American Psychiatric Association, Washington DC, 1994.

Andrews, G., Crino, R., Hunt, C., Lampe, L. and Page, A., *The Treatment of Anxiety Disorders*, Cambridge University Press, Melbourne, 1994.

Beck, A.T., *Cognitive Therapy and the Emotional Disorders*, International Universities Press, New York, 1976.

Booth, A., *Making the Internet Work for your Business*, Allen and Unwin, Sydney, 1999.

Ellis, A. and Harper, R.A., *A New Guide to Rational Living*, Wilshire Book Company, Los Angeles, 1975.

Green, C., *Beyond Toddlerdom – Keeping five to twelve year olds on the rails*, Doubleday, Sydney, 2000.

Greenberger, D. and Padesky, C., *Mind over Mood – Change how you feel by changing the way you think*, Guildford Press, New York, 1995.

Greenfield, D., *Virtual Addiction: Help for netheads, cyberfreaks, and those who love them*, New Harbinger, Oakland, 1999.

Holliday, H., 'Hooked on the Net', *Psychology Today*, 2000, vol. 33, p. 10.

Lamble, J. and Morris, S., *Side by Side: How to think differently about your relationship*, Finch Publishing, Sydney, 2000.

Mitchell, P., 'Internet Addiction: Genuine diagnosis or not?', *The Lancet*, 2000, vol. 355, p. 632.

Rheingold, H., *The Virtual Community – Homesteading on the electronic frontier*, A William Patrick Book, USA, 1993.

Tarbox, K., *Katie.com*, Dutton, New York, 2000.

Wallace, P., *The Psychology of the Internet*, Cambridge University Press, Cambridge, 1999.

Young, K.S., *Caught in the Net: How to recognize the signs of Internet addiction – and a winning strategy for recovery*, John Wiley & Sons, New York, 1998.

Other Finch titles

Chasing Ideas: The fun of freeing your child's imagination
Christine Durham (2001)

This book is a stimulating resource of ideas for parents of children of all ages. Christine Durham has compiled a treasure trove of techniques and tips to help parents with the delightful process of encouraging children's curiosity about the world. *Chasing Ideas* is a fascinating mixture of thinking skills and techniques to help parents unlock their children's minds and give them confidence.

ISBN 1876451 181

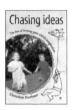

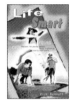

Life Smart: Choices for young people about friendship, family and future
Vicki Bennett (2001)

This important book for teenagers provides a valuable perspective and sound advice on how to deal with the most pressing issues of those vital years – the ups and downs of friendship and love, learning to accept ourselves and others, creating a direction in our lives, and relating to our families.

ISBN 1 876451 130

ParentCraft: A practical guide to raising children well (2nd edition)
Ken and Elizabeth Mellor (2001)

In this practical and commonsense guide (now in its second edition) Ken and Elizabeth Mellor provide important parenting skills and tested ways for parents to deal with a wide range of family situations. They include insights into the cycles and stages of childhood as well as how our family backgrounds contribute to what we do. They explore other themes that relate to managing families, catering for the needs of parents and children, setting standards and limits, love and discipline, and integrating important values into parenting.

ISBN 1876451 19X

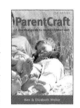

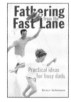

Fathering From the Fast Lane: Practical ideas for busy dads
Dr Bruce Robinson (2001)

The pressures of working life today mean that many fathers are not spending the time with their children that they would like. This book presents practical and straightforward ways to improve this situation. In this collection of valuable fathering ideas, over 75 men from various backgrounds speak about how they balance demanding jobs with being a good dad.

ISBN 1876451 211

Kids Food Health 1: Nutrition and your child's development – the first year
Dr Patricia McVeagh and Eve Reed (2001)

The foods you give your infant form the basis for your child's nutrition and health, now and in the future. The authors specialise in children's health and nutrition, and their experience provides parents with important and reassuring information based on extensive clinical experience and research. Topics covered include: growth problems in the first year; breastfeeding; introducing solids; food allergies and food intolerance; 'Colic'; regurgitation, reflux and vomiting; and dental care.

ISBN 1876451 149

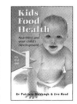

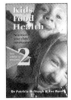

Kids Food Health 2: Nutrition and your child's development – from toddler to preschooler

Dr Patricia McVeagh and Eve Reed (2001)

Children in these years develop assertive independence and have a reputation for being fussy eaters. They know when they are hungry and when they are not. With a few simple rules, good nutrition at this stage is easy. In this book the authors provide straightforward and healthy options for feeding your toddler and preschooler. Topics covered include: normal behaviour and normal eating; the night feeder; dental care; vegetarian eating; food additives; allergies; difficult behaviours; constipation; and not growing well.

ISBN 1876451 157

Kids Food Health 3: Nutrition and your child's development – from school-age to teenage

Dr Patricia McVeagh and Eve Reed (2001)

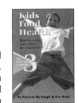

At school, the peer group becomes important in moulding children's food preferences, which are also influenced by the pressures of food advertising. This occurs at an age when some nutrient intakes such as iron and calcium are critical and when serious nutritional problems (including obesity and anorexia nervosa) can occur. In this book the authors aim to guide parents in establishing healthy eating habits that their children will carry into adulthood. Topics covered include: fast food; food additives; food for sport; vegetarian diets; dental care; growth and weight issues; eating disorders; allergies; and food and behaviour.

ISBN 1876451 165

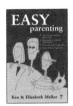

Easy Parenting

Ken and Elizabeth Mellor (2001)

is about meeting the challenges that parents face in raising their children to become well-balanced adults. In a straightforward and accessible style, Ken and Elizabeth Mellor offer many practical skills and approaches, including:

- different ways of loving your child
- using repetition to help children learn
- developing your child's self-esteem
- struggling with children for their benefit
- finding out what your child needs
- getting children to understand what you say
- managing conflicts between siblings
- effective ways to discipline.

ISBN 1876451 114

The Happy Family

Ken and Elizabeth Mellor (2001)

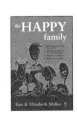

is about how to make family life enjoyable. In this book, Ken and Elizabeth Mellor suggest that our families are little communities in which children learn how to live in the wider world. The authors provide simple, easy-to-use ways to manage our families well. Their practical advice on how to do this includes:

- understanding and changing your family patterns
- creating balance between family life and work
- learning from your childhood experience of families
- handling family conflicts
- working together as a parenting team.

ISBN 1876451 122

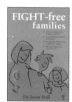

Fight-free Families
Dr Janet Hall (2001)

In *Fight-free Families*, Dr Hall provides solutions to conflicts in a wide range of family situations, from young children through to adolescents. Dr Hall provides proven fight-prevention strategies, ways to resolve fights so everyone wins, and an understanding of what triggers conflict.

ISBN 1876451 22X

Fear-free Children
Dr Janet Hall (2001)

Fear-free Children presents imaginative ways of helping children deal with their fears, such as fear of the dark, fear of animals and fear of being alone. The book draws on real-life case studies to help parents recognise their child's fear symptoms, overcome specific fears and anxieties, and use games to build confidence.

ISBN 1876451 238

Stories of Manhood: Journeys into the hidden hearts of men
Edited by Steve Biddulph (2000)

Steve Biddulph presents his selection of the best writings from around the world on the inner lives of men. By turns powerful, heartrending, wise and funny, these stories are chosen with a single purpose – to break down the narrow stereotypes that men are crushed into.

ISBN 1 876451 106

On Their Own: Boys growing up underfathered
Rex McCann (2000)

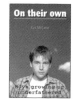

For a young man, the absence of an involved father in his life can create a powerful sense of loss that he takes into adulthood. Such an absence (whether caused by his father's death, divorce, lack of time or interest) can lead to real difficulties in his adult relationships and his role as a parent.

ISBN 1876451 084

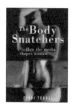

The Body Snatchers: How the media shapes women
Cyndi Tebbel (2000)

There is hardly a woman alive – fat, thin or in-between – who doesn't wish she could alter the body she was born with. From childhood on, women are told they can never be too thin or too young. Cyndi Tebbel exposes the rampant conditioning of women and girls by those pushing starvation imagery, and encourages us to challenge society's preoccupation with an ideal body that is unnatural and (for most) unattainable.

ISBN 1 876451 076

Girls' Talk: Young women speak their hearts and minds
Maria Pallotta-Chiarolli (1998)

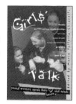

This is the book that every teenage girl should read. Over 150 young women contribute their thoughts and stories on relationships, bodies, families, school life, sex and love, prejudice, feminism and independence.

ISBN 1 876451 025

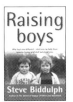

Raising Boys: Why boys are different – and how to help them become happy and well-balanced men
Steve Biddulph (1997)

In his international bestseller, author Steve Biddulph examines the crucial ways that boys differ from girls. He looks at boys' development from birth to manhood and discusses the parenting and guidance boys need.

ISBN 0 646 31418 1

Manhood: An action plan for changing men's lives (2nd edn)
Steve Biddulph (1995)

This bestselling book has had a profound effect on the lives of thousands of men and women around the world. Steve Biddulph discusses issues such as love and sexuality, being a father, finding meaning in work, making real friends and forming new partnerships with women.

ISBN 0 646261 44 4

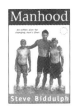

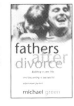

Beginning Fatherhood: A guide for expectant fathers
Warwick Pudney and Judy Cottrell. (1998)

A warm and informative book for the man about to start the most important job of his life. It is full of practical and commonsense advice and encourages men to be active partners in the birth process.

ISBN 1 876451 01 7

Fathers After Divorce: Building a new life and becoming a successful separated father
Michael Green (1998)

This practical handbook includes straightforward checklists for separated fathers to use in overcoming problems and developing a positive outlook, as well as advice from many men on how to begin a new life.

ISBN 1 876451 00 9

Dealing with Anger: Self-help solutions for men
Frank Donovan (1999)

This book aims to help men solve their anger problems and eliminate the risk of anger-driven violence. A step-by-step program focuses on emotional healing, behaviour control and practical change.

ISBN 1 876451 05X

Boys in Schools: Addressing the real issues – behaviour, values and relationships
Rollo Browne & Richard Fletcher (eds) (1995)

Fifteen classroom teachers, from primary and secondary schools, provide positive accounts of how they changed boys' behaviour to improve learning, relationships and the whole school environment.

ISBN 0 646 239589

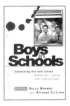

Other books by Jo Lamble and Sue Morris

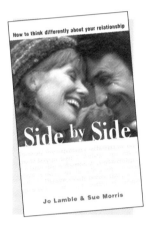

Side by Side: How to think differently about your relationship

The authors provide strategies for individuals and couples to identify and overcome common relationship problems, to help them communicate better with their partners and consider issues such as their expectations, commitment and attitude to their partner's qualities.

Jo Lamble and Sue Morris (2000)
ISBN 1876451 092

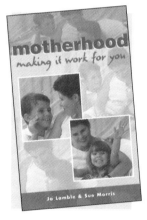

Motherhood: Making it work for you

At times, many mothers may feel that their lives are out of control. *Motherhood* is designed to help women deal with the pressures of family life and the expectations of being a mum of children of all ages.

Jo Lamble & Sue Morris (1999)
ISBN 1 876451 033

Jo Lamble and Sue Morris can be contacted at lamblemorris@bigpond.com

---

FINCH

Publishers of books on parenting, relationships and social issues

Contact Finch Publishing

To see our latest titles or contact our authors, visit our website: www.finch.com.au. Finch titles are available in bookshops throughout Australia, New Zealand, South Africa and many countries in Asia. Alternatively write to us at P O Box 120, Lane Cove 1595, Australia. Phone (02) 9418 6247 Fax (02) 9418 8878.

Index